Rheumatology

A Clinical Handbook

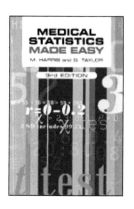
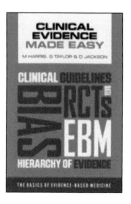
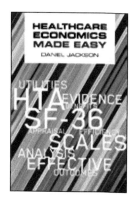
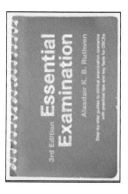
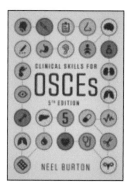
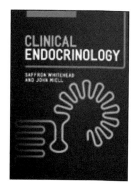
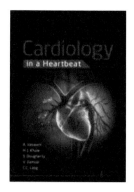
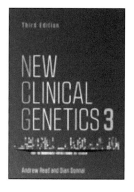
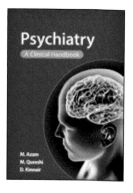
For more details see www.scionpublishing.com

Rheumatology

A Clinical Handbook

Ahmad Al-Sukaini & Mohsin Azam
University of Leicester

Ash Samanta
Consultant Rheumatologist, University Hospitals of Leicester NHS Trust

Scion

A CIP catalogue record for this book is available from the British Library.

ISBN 978 1 907904 26 4

Scion Publishing Limited

The Old Hayloft, Vantage Business Park, Bloxham Road, Banbury OX16 9UX, UK

www.scionpublishing.com

Important Note from the Publisher

The information contained within this book was obtained by Scion Publishing Ltd from sources believed by us to be reliable. However, while every effort has been made to ensure its accuracy, no responsibility for loss or injury whatsoever occasioned to any person acting or refraining from action as a result of information contained herein can be accepted by the authors or publishers.

Readers are reminded that medicine is a constantly evolving science and while the authors and publishers have ensured that all dosages, applications and practices are based on current indications, there may be specific practices which differ between communities. You should always follow the guidelines laid down by the manufacturers of specific products and the relevant authorities in the country in which you are practising.

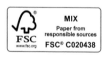
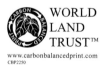

www.carbonbalancedprint.com
CBP2250

Line artwork by Hilary Strickland Illustration, Bath, UK

Typeset by Medlar Publishing Solutions Pvt Ltd, India

Printed in the UK

Contents

Preface vii
Acknowledgments viii
Abbreviations ix

1   Introduction 1

2   Specific conditions 7
   2.1 Rheumatoid arthritis 8
   2.2 Osteoarthritis 14
   2.3 Septic arthritis 19
       Introduction to spondyloarthropathies 22
   2.4 Psoriatic arthritis 23
   2.5 Ankylosing spondylitis 27
   2.6 Reactive arthritis 31
   2.7 Gout 35
   2.8 Calcium pyrophosphate disease 39
   2.9 Vasculitis 41
   2.10 Giant cell arteritis 48
   2.11 Polymyalgia rheumatica 52
   2.12 Systemic lupus erythematosus 55
   2.13 Polymyositis and dermatomyositis 61
   2.14 Sjögren's syndrome 65
   2.15 Scleroderma 68
   2.16 Fibromyalgia 73
   2.17 Osteoporosis 76
   2.18 Paget's disease 81

3   Paediatric rheumatology conditions 85
   3.1 Vitamin D deficiency 86
   3.2 Juvenile idiopathic arthritis 91

4   Investigations 97
   4.1 Blood tests 98
   4.2 Immunological tests 103
   4.3 Synovial fluid analysis 106
   4.4 Imaging 108

5 Pharmacology 111

   5.1   Analgesia 112

   5.2   Corticosteroids 116

   5.3   Osteoporosis drugs 118

   5.4   DMARDs and biological agents 122

6 OSCEs 129

   6.1   History taking 130

   6.2   Examination 133

   6.3   Differential diagnosis 138

Appendix A   Answers to self-assessment questions 141

Appendix B   Photograph acknowledgments 147

Index 151

Additional self-assessment questions are available from:

www.scionpublishing.com/rheumatologyQandA

Preface

In my experience of teaching rheumatology at undergraduate (and postgraduate) level for over thirty years, there is one consistent response that I have come across from medical students. This is a general fear of rheumatology. The reason many students regard rheumatology as mysterious and arcane is because of a lack of understanding about what rheumatology covers, as well as a somewhat fuzzy knowledge of the various conditions that are encompassed within rheumatology.

Some years ago I thought it might be helpful for medical students (at the University of Leicester) if I put together what I termed 'revision notes' for rheumatology. I would often encourage students to offer any suggestions for change but the reality was that no-one ever did. A couple of years ago, two bright young medical students, Ahmad Al-Sukaini and Mohsin Azam (who are co-authors of this text) approached me after one of my lectures and came up with a number of ideas, and the revision notes were updated in due course. They also suggested putting together a short book that would be more comprehensive than just brief notes, and that would flag key issues in rheumatology for undergraduate medical students. Their enthusiasm, effort and assistance are to be strongly commended.

According to surveys we carried out at the University of Leicester, students wholeheartedly agreed that a rheumatology 'guide' would be of benefit to them and to junior doctors. Their preference was to use bullet point formatting and an approach that would be succinct and highly focused, as opposed to the more conventional paragraphs and narrative writing. We have also used a wide range of pedagogic features, including summary tables, illustrations and mnemonics throughout. Furthermore, the size of the book was important – it had to be one that could be carried around easily. To test student knowledge and reinforce learning, questions were devised within the framework used by examiners. Single Best Answer (SBA) and Extended Matching Questions (EMQs) are increasingly being utilized by medical school examiners to explore understanding of a topic and it is essential that students familiarize themselves with these types of question. The questions, together with their answers, can be found online, as mentioned at the end of the Contents.

We took up this challenge and have put together this text with the aim of covering rheumatology in a clear and concise manner. The content thoroughly encompasses the current medical school curriculum in the UK and we hope that this text will be highly beneficial to medical students for furthering their knowledge, as well as a revision guide for undergraduate examination purposes. We also hope that it will assist newly qualified junior doctors and serve as a quick reference guide for clinics and ward-based work. The concise and coherent format of this book is likely to appeal to other healthcare professionals who require a working knowledge of rheumatology.

Finally, I would say that this text is not intended to replace any of the standard erudite text books in rheumatology that have already been published. It is designed to focus the mind, provide concise guidance, and encourage further exploration of rheumatology.

Dr Ash Samanta
Consultant Rheumatologist, University of Leicester
January 2014

Acknowledgments

We are extremely grateful to the medical students of the University of Leicester who gave invaluable advice on the content and structure of the text. We are also very grateful to Dr Rebecca Neame for her help in conducting the student survey. Our deepest appreciation goes to Dr Parthajit Das, Dr Shireen Shaffu and Dr Kenny Sunmboye for their contribution to the SBA and EMQ questions. We would also like to sincerely thank our friend Adeel Qureshi for sharing his remarkable experience in market research with us.

We would also like to place on record our sincere gratitude to the team at Scion Publishing Ltd, particularly Dr Jonathan Ray and Ms Clare Boomer, for their great support, encouragement and patience.

Please refer to Appendix B for acknowledgment to the copyright holders of the many images in the book.

Dedications

To my parents and family for all the unconditional love and support they have for me.
Thank you for your unfailing faith and enthusiasm.
Special thanks go to my uncle, Sabah, for being a truly inspirational person to me. You have been my mentor and a great blessing.   A.A.

To the memory of my loving grandparents who always believed in me. I will always treasure the priceless memories we shared together.
My deepest appreciation goes to my parents and the rest of my family. Without your continued support and inspiration, none of this would have been possible.   M.A.

For my 'long-suffering' family.   A.S.

Abbreviations

ACA	anti-centromere antibody	FBC	full blood count
ACE	angiotension-converting enzyme	FRAX	Fracture Risk Assessment Tool
ACR	American College of Rheumatology	FSH	follicle-stimulating hormone
		GBM	glomerular basement disease
ALP	alkaline phosphatase	GCA	giant cell arteritis
ANA	antinuclear antibodies	GI	gastrointestinal
ANCA	antineutrophil cytoplasmic antibodies	GORD	gastro-oesophageal reflux disease
ARF	acute renal failure	GPA	granulomatous polyangiitis
AS	ankylosing spondylitis	GU	genitourinary
BMD	bone mineral density	HAART	highly active antiretroviral treatment
BMI	body mass index	Hb	haemoglobin
BP	blood pressure	HBV	hepatitis B virus
CBT	cognitive behavioural therapy	HLA	human leucocyte antigen
CCF	congestive cardiac failure	HRT	hormone replacement therapy
CCP	cyclic citrullinated peptide	HSP	Henoch–Schönlein purpura
CK	creatine kinase	IBD	inflammatory bowel disease
CNS	central nervous system	IHD	ischaemic heart disease
CPPD	calcium pyrophosphate disease	IL	interleukin
CRP	C-reactive protein	ILAR	International League of Associations for Rheumatology
CSS	Churg–Strauss syndrome		
CT	computerized tomography	IV	intravenous
CVS	cardiovascular system	JIA	juvenile idiopathic arthritis
CXR	chest X-ray	JRA	juvenile rheumatoid arthritis
DAS	Disease Activity Score	LDH	lactate dehydrogenase
DEXA	dual-energy X-ray absorptiometry	LFT	liver function test
		MCP	metacarpophalangeal
DIP	distal interphalangeal	MCTD	mixed connective tissue disease
DM	dermatomyositis		
DMARD	disease-modifying antirheumatic drug	MI	myocardial infarction
		MMP	metalloprotease
DNA	deoxyribonucleic acid	MPA	microscopic polyangiitis
DVT	deep vein thrombosis	MRI	magnetic resonance imaging
ECG	electrocardiogram	MSK	musculoskeletal
EDTA	ethylenediaminetetraacetic acid	MSU	monosodium urate
		MTP	metatarso-phalangeal
EMG	electromyography	NICE	National Institute for Health and Care Excellence
ERA	endothelin-1 receptor antagonists		
		NSAID	non-steroidal anti-inflammatory drug
ESR	erythrocyte sedimentation rate		
EULAR	European League Against Rheumatism	OA	osteoarthritis
		PAN	polyarteritis nodosa

PCV	packed cell volume	SpA	spondyloarthropathy
PDE	phosphodiesterase	SS	Sjögren's syndrome
PIP	proximal interphalangeal	SSc	systemic sclerosis
PM	polymyositis	SUA	serum uric acid
PMR	polymyalgia rheumatica	TB	tuberculosis
PPI	proton pump inhibitor	TFT	thyroid function test
PsA	psoriatic arthritis	TNF	tumour necrosis factor
PTH	parathyroid hormone	USS	ultrasound scan
RA	rheumatoid arthritis	UTI	urinary tract infection
RF	rheumatoid factor	VTE	venous thromboembolism
RFT	renal function test	WCC	white cell count
ROS	reactive oxygen species	WG	Wegener's granulomatosis
SI	sacroiliac	WHO	World Health Organization
SLE	systemic lupus erythematosus		

Chapter 1

Introduction

What is rheumatology?

Rheumatology is a multidisciplinary branch of medicine that encompasses the investigation, diagnosis and management of patients with arthritis and other musculoskeletal conditions. This includes many disorders affecting joints, bones, muscles and soft tissues. A significant number of musculoskeletal conditions also affect other organ systems and occur as part of a systemic autoimmune disease. The main rheumatological disorders are summarized in *Fig. 1.1* and will be covered in significant depth.

The rheumatology multidisciplinary team (MDT) consists of a variety of disciplines that work together with the aim of providing optimal care to sufferers via a holistic approach (*Fig. 1.2*). The team consists of many healthcare professionals including consultant rheumatologists, general practitioners (GPs), occupational therapists, orthopaedic surgeons, physiotherapists, psychiatrists, special nurses and many more.

Rheumatologists are specialists who deal with a wide range of rheumatic diseases. They assess overall function, including physical and mental wellbeing and level of independence. They also manage results of advanced imaging and lab tests, treatment options and the need for further assessment and management, such as referrals to other healthcare providers.

Outline of the book

Chapter 2

For each condition the following will be covered:

- **Pathophysiology**: the information surrounding the pathophysiology of rheumatology disorders is constantly evolving and there is still so much that remains to be understood. Up-to-date resources were used with the intention of keeping this section simple and concise and not overlooking the clinical aspects of rheumatology!

- **Epidemiology and risk factors**: attention has been paid to the incidence / prevalence of the rheumatology disorders so that students are aware of the very common, less common and rare disorders. Where possible, risk factors are arranged in a descending order of importance via a simple to follow table, to highlight the most important risk factors for students to learn.

- **Clinical features**: a variety of pedagogical features such as X-rays, photographs and illustrations have been used, as well as **red flags** indicated by, and mnemonics in green. Red flags or alarm systems refer to symptoms which are suggestive of significant pathology and should therefore not be missed or neglected. These devices are aimed at enabling students to have a greater understanding of the features to look out for and also as an aid to information retention.

- **Diagnosis and investigations**: this element is centred on the diagnostic pathway – history taking, physical examination, investigations and possible differential diagnoses. It is conveyed in an easy to follow box format. Wherever relevant, up-to-date clinical guidelines, including those from the National Institute for Health and Care Excellence (NICE), the European League Against Rheumatism (EULAR) and the American College of Rheumatology (ACR), were utilized. *Chapter 4* has also been created specifically for investigations, to provide further detail of the various tests performed in rheumatology.

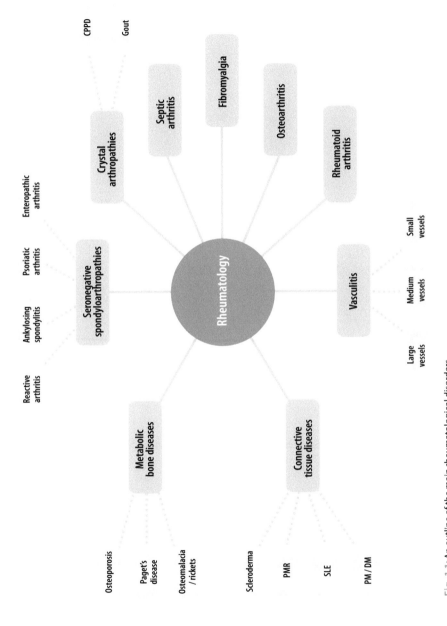

Fig. 1.1: An outline of the main rheumatological disorders.

- ***Management***: this part also utilizes clinical guidelines. Flowcharts, tables and diagrams are used to convey information more effectively and render it more memorable. *Chapter 5* covers the main pharmacological agents of rheumatology in further detail.

- **OSCE tip / rapid diagnosis / clinical fact box:**   wherever applicable, extra information is provided in the form of tips for the OSCE examination, empirical diagnostic features to form a 'rapid diagnosis' and important clinical facts for students to be aware of.

Self-assessment questions conclude each specific condition section. These are designed for students to check that they have understood and grasped the material.

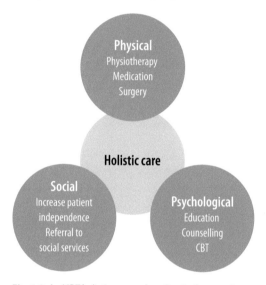

Fig. 1.2: An MDT holistic approach outline to rheumatology.

Chapter 3

This chapter consists of two important and common conditions in rheumatology which present during early life: vitamin D deficiency including both rickets and osteomalacia and juvenile idiopathic arthritis. The same longitudinal format is used as above.

Chapter 4

It may be advisable to read this before embarking on the main rheumatological conditions text (*Chapter 2*), as it provides a basic understanding of the three principal investigations used in rheumatology to reach a definitive diagnosis: blood tests, imaging and synovial fluid analysis.

Chapter 5

This should be used as a cross-reference with *Chapter 2*, in order for students to gain a deeper understanding of the way in which pharmacological agents work, as well as the side-effects and contraindications. It provides information about commonly used agents including analgesics, corticosteroids, osteoporosis agents, DMARDs and biological agents. This section also includes '**DO**' and '**DO NOT**' boxes so that students are aware of the essentials and common pitfalls, respectively, when prescribing pharmacological agents.

Chapter 6

This focuses on the key points of history taking and performing clinical examinations, with particular emphasis on the GALS and hand examination, so that students have a thorough structure to follow and therefore do not panic when it comes to the dreaded OSCE examinations!

In order to make the book more affordable, additional questions in the form of single best answer questions (SBAs) and extended matching questions (EMQs) have been made available online as a free resource to complement the material in the book. To access the questions and answers, go to www.scionpublishing.com/rheumatologyQandA

Chapter 2

Specific conditions

2.1	Rheumatoid arthritis	8
2.2	Osteoarthritis	14
2.3	Septic arthritis	19
	Introduction to spondyloarthropathies	22
2.4	Psoriatic arthritis	23
2.5	Ankylosing spondylitis	27
2.6	Reactive arthritis	31
2.7	Gout	35
2.8	Calcium pyrophosphate disease	39
2.9	Vasculitis	41
2.10	Giant cell arteritis	48
2.11	Polymyalgia rheumatica	52
2.12	Systemic lupus erythematosus	55
2.13	Polymyositis and dermatomyositis	61
2.14	Sjögren's syndrome	65
2.15	Scleroderma	68
2.16	Fibromyalgia	73
2.17	Osteoporosis	76
2.18	Paget's disease	81

2.1 Rheumatoid arthritis

Rheumatoid arthritis (RA) is a **chronic systemic inflammatory** disorder which primarily affects joints that are lined with **synovium**. It is typically characterized by a **symmetrical**, occasionally **deforming**, **peripheral polyarthritis**. Because it is a **systemic disease**, it can also affect the whole body, including the heart, lungs and eyes.

Pathophysiology

- The actual cause of RA is not entirely understood.
- It is likely that **genetically susceptible** individuals are exposed to an unknown antigen resulting in self-stimulation of the immune system **(autoimmunity)**.
- The immune response cross-reacts with the **host tissue (synovial membrane)** resulting in **inflammation** of the **synovial membrane (synovitis)** that lines **joints** and **tendon sheaths**. This gives rise to **synovial hypertrophy**.
- This process can eventually lead to **cartilage damage** and **bone destruction**.
- **T-cells** seem to be the most important mediators of the disease. They stimulate the immune system via the release of a variety of **inflammatory cytokines**, most importantly **TNF-α**, **IL-1** and **IL-6**, resulting in a **pro-inflammatory state** (*Fig. 2.1.1*).

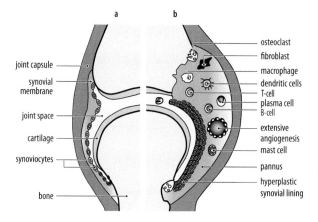

Fig. 2.1.1: (a) Normal healthy joint with thin synovial membrane and **(b)** an RA joint. Various inflammatory cells, such as T-cells, macrophages and plasma cells infiltrate the synovial membrane to make it hyperplastic. Ultimately it develops into a 'pannus' which migrates onto and into articular cartilage and underlying bone.

Epidemiology and risk factors

- **Prevalence**: there are approximately 400 000 people with RA in the UK.
- **Incidence**: approximately 20 000 people are diagnosed with new RA each year in the UK.
- Certain risk factors have been linked to RA (*Table 2.1.1*).

Table 2.1.1: Risk factors for RA	
Gender	• **Before menopause**, RA is **3 times** more common in **women** than men; **after** menopause the distribution is similar.
Age	• Rheumatoid arthritis can affect any age group but the age of onset is often **20–40 years**.
Familial	• Estimated to account for **60%** of disease susceptibility.
Genetic	• There are strong associations between **HLA-DR4 and HLA-DR1** and RA, which may be **familial or non-familial (sporadic)**.
Environmental factors	• **Smoking**, infection, diet and hormonal.

Clinical features

The **S** factor:

1. **S**tiffness in the morning >1 hour
2. **S**ymmetrical joint pain
3. **S**wollen joints (polyarthritis)
4. **S**mall joints of the hand, feet and wrist (mainly affected)
5. **S**ex: female:male ratio is 3:1
6. **S**peed: quick onset over weeks to months
7. **S**pecific signs for the hand:
   a. *Early*: swollen metacarpophalangeal (MCP), proximal interphalangeal (PIP), wrist or metatarso-phalangeal (MTP) joints.
   b. *Later* (*Fig. 2.1.2a*): **Boutonnière deformity** (flexion of the PIP and hyperextension of the distal interphalangeal (DIP) joints), **swan neck deformity** (hyperextension of PIP and flexion of DIP joints), Z-thumb (hyperextension of the interphalangeal joint, and fixed flexion and subluxation of the MCP joint) and **ulnar deviation** (subluxation of proximal phalanges towards the ulnar side).
8. **S**everal extra-articular manifestations (*Fig. 2.1.3*).

a

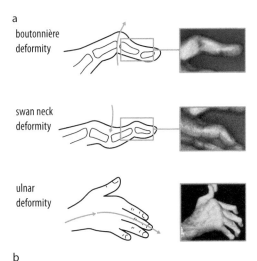

boutonnière deformity

swan neck deformity

ulnar deformity

b

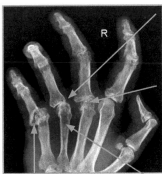

Narrowing of joint space

Juxta-articular bone erosion

Subluxation of proximal phalanx

Periarticular osteopenia

Fig. 2.1.2: (a) Late specific signs of RA; (b) Late X-ray features of RA.

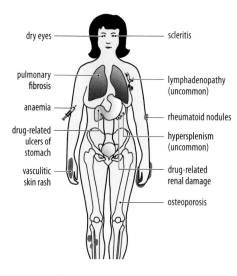

dry eyes

scleritis

pulmonary fibrosis

lymphadenopathy (uncommon)

anaemia

rheumatoid nodules

drug-related ulcers of stomach

hypersplenism (uncommon)

vasculitic skin rash

drug-related renal damage

osteoporosis

OSCE tips: RA vs OA clinical features!

- **RA** usually presents symmetrically, osteoarthritis (**OA**) usually presents with asymmetrical joint pain
- **RA** morning stiffness >1 hour, **OA** <30 minutes
- OA is worse on movement, RA is not
- Common age of onset for **RA** is 20–40 years and >50 years for **OA**
- **RA** onset is relatively rapid (weeks to months), **OA** typically years
- **RA** presents with systemic symptoms, **OA** doesn't
- **RA** tends to be worse in the morning, **OA** is worse after activities, especially towards the end of the day

Fig. 2.1.3: The extra-articular manifestations of the disease can occur at any age after onset and occur more commonly in males despite RA being more common in females. Extra-articular organs may involve the skin, eyes, heart, lungs and kidneys.

Diagnosis and investigations (see *Table 2.1.2*)

All people suspected of having RA should be referred for specialist assessment.

	Diagnosis	Prognostic indicators
Hx	• Pain duration (usually ≥6 weeks), morning stiffness >1 hour	• Activity limitations, comorbidities, risk factors such as smoking and family history
Ex	• ≥3 swollen tender joints, symmetrical joint involvement, subcutaneous nodules	• Extra-articular manifestations (*Fig. 2.1.3*)
Ix	• ↑ **Serum rheumatoid factor (RF)** • ↑ **Anti-cyclic citrullinated peptide antibodies (anti-CCP)** • ↑ **Erythrocyte sedimentation rate (ESR) / C-reactive protein (CRP)** **Note:** *RF has ↑ sensitivity and ↓ specificity; anti-CCP has ↑ specificity and ↓ sensitivity*	• **Full blood count**: ↑ platelet count, ↑ serum ferritin, anaemia of chronic disease • **Renal and liver function tests** • **X-ray**: chest, hands (*Fig. 2.1.2b*) and feet • **MRI**: identify synovitis early • **Ultrasound**: joint effusion and Baker's cysts
DDx	• Psoriatic arthritis • Connective tissue disease, e.g. systemic lupus erythematosus (SLE)	• Reactive arthritis • Polymyalgia rheumatica

Table 2.1.2: The 2010 American College of Rheumatology (ACR) and the European League against Rheumatism (EULAR) criteria

The most recent criteria for the diagnosis of RA are the 2010 ACR and the EULAR criteria. A total score of ≥6 is diagnostic of RA.	Score
A. Joint involvement:	
1 large joint	0
2–10 large joints	1
1–3 small joints (with or without involvement of large joints)	2
4–10 small joints (with or without involvement of large joints)	3
B. Serology:	
Negative RF and negative anti-CCP	0
Low-positive RF or low-positive anti-CCP	2
High-positive RF or high-positive anti-CCP	3
C. Acute phase reactants:	
Normal CRP and normal ESR	0
Abnormal CRP or abnormal ESR	1
D. Duration of symptoms:	
<6 weeks	0
≥6 weeks	1

Note: The 2010 EULAR and ACR criteria replaced the 1987 ACR criteria as they focus on features at an earlier stage of the disease that are associated with persistent and/or erosive disease, rather than defining the disease by its late-stage features. As a result, this refocuses attention on the important need for earlier diagnosis and therefore earlier treatment.

Management

The aim of management in RA is to reduce / slow the joint inflammation and disease progression to maintain the patient's lifestyle. Early use of **disease-modifying antirheumatic drugs (DMARDs)** and **biological agents** improves the long-term outcome of the disease. Treatment should be started **within 3 months** of symptom onset, based on NICE CG79 (2009).

- Refer urgently to a **rheumatologist**, in order to prevent irreversible destruction of joint(s) if:
  - the **small joints of the hand and feet** are affected
  - more than one joint is affected
  - there has been a delay of 3 months or longer between the onset of symptoms and seeking medical advice.
- Specialists usually start with a **DMARD and short-term corticosteroids** (if appropriate). Emphasis should be placed on reaching a clinical effective dose rather than on the choice of DMARD.
- The disease activity of RA should be monitored by measuring **CRP** and the **DAS28 score** (*Box 2.1.1*). The aim is to reduce the **DAS28 score below 3**.

Non-pharmacological management

- Encourage regular exercise: aerobic activities, flexibility and muscle strength exercises, **core stability exercise**, **balance rehabilitation**, promotion of lifestyle physical activity, smoking cessation.
- People with RA should have access to a **multidisciplinary team** such as **specialist nurses**, **physiotherapists, occupational therapists and podiatrists**.

Table 2.1.3: Pharmacological management of rheumatoid arthritis

DMARDs	• Are **first-line** • Early DMARD treatment is associated with better long-term prognosis. Ideally within 3 months of the onset of persistent symptoms • **Methotrexate, sulfasalazine** and **hydroxychloroquine** are the most commonly used • NICE recommends a combination of DMARDs, including methotrexate and at least one other DMARD, plus short-term glucocorticoids (if not contraindicated)
Corticosteroids	• Rapid reduction in **symptom onset** and **inflammation** • Can be given via **intra-muscular, intra-articular** and **oral routes** • NICE recommends a combination of corticosteroids and DMARDs
NSAIDs	For **symptomatic relief** and also to **reduce inflammation**, e.g. **ibuprofen, diclofenac, etodolac**
Biological agents (TNF-α inhibitors, B-cell blockers, and anti-IL-1 & IL-6 agents). Indications: after the failure of 2 conventional non-biological DMARDs. Failure is measured objectively using DAS28 (indicated by a score >5.1)	
TNF-α inhibitors	• Block the pivotal action of TNF-α, a key cytokine in the pathogenesis of RA • Include **infliximab, adalimumab** and **etanercept** • Very **expensive** and used in **severe cases (high DAS28 score)** • Should normally be used in combination with methotrexate
B-cell blockers	• **Rituximab** is a **B-cell blocker** • It works by targeting the **B-cell surface marker, CD-20** • A combination of **rituximab** and **methotrexate** is recommended as an option for the treatment of adults with RA who are intolerant of other DMARDs or whose response to them is inadequate.
Anti IL-1 & IL-6 agents	• Like TNF- α, IL-1 and IL-6 are pro-inflammatory cytokines which are heavily involved in the disease process. • **Anakinra** is an **IL-1 receptor antagonist** • **Tocilizumab** is an **anti-IL-6 receptor monoclonal antibody** • On the balance of its clinical benefits and cost-effectiveness, anakinra is not recommended for the treatment of rheumatoid arthritis

Pharmacological: see *Table 2.1.3*

Surgery:

- Consider the following for surgical opinion if they do not respond to non-surgical management:
  - **Persistent pain** due to joint damage or other identifiable soft tissue cause
  - **Worsening joint function**
  - **Progressive deformity**
  - **Persistent localized synovitis**.
- Surgical procedures may include:
  - **Joint prosthesis**: **hip** and **knee**
  - **Arthroscopy**: remove abnormal synovium, cartilage and eroded bone
  - **Tendon reconstruction**: restore function when tendon ruptured.

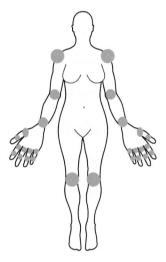

Box 2.1.1: The Disease Activity Score (DAS)28

- It assesses **tenderness and swelling at 28 joints** (see *Fig. 2.1.4*), **ESR**, and patients' **self-reported symptom** severity, to calculate a disease activity score.
  DAS28 score of:
  >5.1 = **high disease activity**
  3.2–5.1 = **moderate disease activity**
  <3.2 = **low disease activity**
  <2.6 = **remission**
- *A decrease in DAS28 score by*:
  0.6 points or less = poor response
  >1.2 points = moderate or good response
  (depending on whether an individual's DAS28 score at the end point is above or below 3.2, respectively)

Fig. 2.1.4: The 28 joints (MCPs, PIPs, wrists, elbows, shoulders and knees) that are examined in calculating DAS28.

Self-assessment

A 45 year old woman complains of symmetrical pain and swelling of her MCP joints. You think that a diagnosis of RA is likely.

1. What clinical features would suggest a diagnosis of RA in this lady?
2. What specific questions would you like to ask her?
3. What blood tests would you initially perform, and what might they show?
4. The blood tests confirm a diagnosis of RA. Which group of pharmacological agents would you use to start specific treatment? Name the most commonly used drugs in this group and their main side-effects.
5. Name two ways of monitoring response to treatment.

Answers to self-assessment questions are to be found in *Appendix A*.

Osteoarthritis

Osteoarthritis (OA) is the **most common form of arthritis** and is a major cause of **impaired mobility**. It is a condition characterized by **cartilage damage** and **joint space narrowing** resulting in **pain**, **functional limitation** and **impaired quality of life**. It can affect any joint but the **hip**, **knee**, **lumbar** or **cervical spine**, and **wrist joints** are most commonly affected.

Pathophysiology

- OA is viewed as a **metabolically dynamic process** where there is an imbalance between joint breakdown and sufficient repair process.
- Normal joint articulating cartilage, **hyaline cartilage**, undergoes turnover in which 'worn out' collagen and other matrix components are degraded and replaced by **chondrocyte cells**.
- Both **genetic and environmental** factors can stimulate **apoptosis** of chondrocytes, disrupting the normal repair mechanism and thereby causing cartilage damage.
- Certain **cytokines** (e.g. **IL-1** and **TNF-α**) and **protease enzymes** (e.g. **metalloproteinase**) increase in the cartilage; this triggers osteoarthritic changes through direct cartilage damage.
- Eventually, cartilage destruction exposes underlying bone, resulting in abnormal **subchondral bone growth (subchondral sclerosis)**, **osteophytes** and **bone cysts** (*Fig. 2.2.1*).

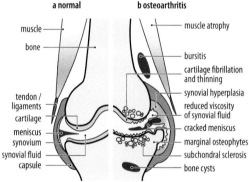

Fig. 2.2.1: **(a)** normal joint **(b)** OA joint.

Epidemiology and risk factors

- Worldwide estimates indicate that 9.6% of men and 18% of women ≥60 years have symptomatic OA.
- At least 4.4 million, 550 000 and 210 000 people in the UK have X-ray evidence of moderate to severe OA of the hands, knees and hips, respectively.

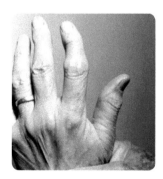

Fig. 2.2.2: Bony enlargements of the DIP joints (Heberden's nodes) and PIP joints (Bouchard's nodes) due to osteophyte formation.

Table 2.2.1: Risk factors for OA

Systemic risk factors		Mechanical risk factors	
Age	• Risk increases with age; partly due to age-related changes such as ligament laxity.	**Obesity**	• Places mechanical stress on joint cartilage.
Gender	• Polyarticular OA is more common in women. • A high prevalence in post-menopausal women suggests a role for sex hormones.	**Injury**	• Ligament damage or fractures can lead to abnormal stress on joint cartilage.
		Joint damage	• Joint damage due to underlying disease e.g. RA, Paget's disease, varus and valgus deformity or trauma (secondary OA).
Family history	• 40–60% of 'common OA' is thought to have a hereditary component.	**Joint site**	• Weight-bearing joints are at higher risk.
Bone density	• ↑ bone density e.g. Paget's disease ↑ risk of OA. • ↓ bone density e.g. osteoporosis ↓ risk of OA.	**Occupa-tion**	• Cleaners have ↑ risk of hip, knee and shoulder OA. • Hairdressers have ↑ risk of hand OA. • Farmers have ↑ risk of hip OA.

Clinical features

- Clinical features depend on the joint sites affected (*Table 2.2.2*).

  Symptoms: **Joint pain** – worse on movement, load bearing and at the end of the day, **joint stiffness** – in the morning or after rest for <30 minutes, **reduced joint function** and **joint instability**.

  Signs: **Periarticular tenderness**, **crepitus**, ↓ range of movement, **muscle wasting**, **joint deformity** and **instability**, squaring of the thumb, swelling of the hands (**Bouchard's nodes** and **Heberden's nodes**; *Fig. 2.2.2*), mild **synovitis** and **effusion**.

Table 2.2.2: American College of Rheumatology (ACR) criteria for hand, hip and knee OA

Nodal OA	Nodal OA or primary generalized OA commonly affects post-menopausal women. There is hand pain, aching, or stiffness for most days of the prior month. Heberden's and Bouchard's nodes in ≥2 joints are characteristic of nodal OA.
Hip OA	Hip pain for most days of the prior month. Categorized largely radiographically: femoral and / or acetabular osteophytes and radiograph hip joint-space narrowing.
Knee OA	Commonly presents in obese women ≥38 years of age. There is knee pain for most days of the prior month, crepitus on movement, morning stiffness ≤30 minutes and bony enlargement of the knee on examination.

Diagnosis and investigations

Hx
- **Joint pain** (worsened by exercise & relieved by rest) and **stiffness** (morning / after rest).
- **Reduced joint function** and **joint instability**.
- Ask about **risk factors** e.g. family history and trauma.

Ex
- **Look** → pain on movement, muscle wasting and limp/antalgic gait.
- **Feel** → periarticular tenderness, swelling of joints, mild synovitis and effusion, and absence of systemic features, e.g. fever.
- **Move** → pain on movement, ↓ range of movement, joint deformity, joint instability and crepitus.

Ix
- **Blood tests**: ESR and CRP are usually normal, RF and anti-CCP negative.
- **X-ray ('LOSS')**: **L**oss of joint space, **O**steophytes, **S**ubchondral sclerosis, **S**ubchondral cysts (*Figs. 2.2.3* and *2.2.4*).
- **MRI**: can demonstrate early thinning of cartilage.
- **Arthroscopy**: cartilage loss and erosion.
- **Joint aspiration**: sterile, viscous fluid; white cell count (WCC) may be slightly elevated.

DDx
Large joint involvement:
- Monoarticular inflammatory arthropathy
- Chronic infection e.g. tuberculosis
- Calcium pyrophosphate disease (CPPD) (if knee is involved)

Small polyarticular joint involvement:
- RA

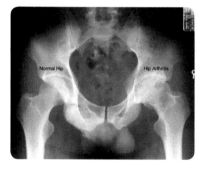

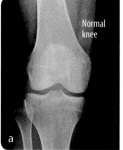

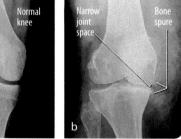

Fig. 2.2.3: X-ray of an individual with a normal right hip and a left hip with OA demonstrating reduced joint space, subchondral cysts and subchondral sclerosis.

Fig. 2.2.4: X-ray of **(a)** a normal joint and **(b)** X-ray of an osteoarthritic knee which shows reduced joint space and bony spurs (osteophytes).

- **Presenting complaint** → Joint pain worse on exercise or after rest? Morning stiffness? Slow timing of onset? Reduced joint function and stability? Weight-bearing joint(s)? Particular joint(s) that is 'overused'?
- **Predisposing factors** → e.g. trauma?
- **Past medical history** → Secondary causes e.g. RA and Paget's disease?
- **Family history** → Family history of OA?
- **Social history** → Occupation?

Management (NICE guidelines, 2014)

- Management of OA includes non-pharmacological management (*Table 2.2.3*), pharmacological pain relief (*Fig. 2.2.5*) and surgical intervention.

Table 2.2.3: Non-pharmacological management of OA	
Education and advice	Education, advice and access to information are core treatments which should be offered to everyone with OA.
Exercise	Exercise should be a core treatment for people with OA and should consist of local muscle strengthening and general aerobic fitness.
Weight loss	Should be a core treatment for OA individuals who are obese or overweight.
Transcutaneous nerve stimulation	A method of electrical stimulation to provide a degree of pain relief. Can be used as an adjunct to core treatment for pain relief.
Aids and devices	Advice on appropriate footwear should be given as part of core treatment for people with lower limb osteoarthritis. People with biomechanical joint pain or instability should be considered for bracing / joint supports / insoles as an adjunct to their core treatment.
Physiotherapy	Can be useful for some individuals with OA.

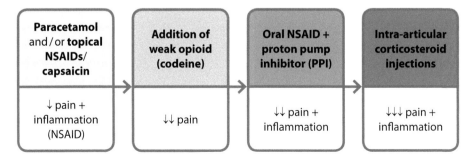

Paracetamol and / or **topical NSAIDs/ capsaicin**	**Addition of weak opioid (codeine)**	**Oral NSAID + proton pump inhibitor (PPI)**	**Intra-articular corticosteroid injections**
↓ pain + inflammation (NSAID)	↓↓ pain	↓↓ pain + inflammation	↓↓↓ pain + inflammation

Fig. 2.2.5: Pharmacological management of OA.

- Surgical intervention is indicated when joint symptoms have a substantial impact on the patient's quality of life and medical management has failed:
  - **Replacement of joint** – the most common operations are to replace hip, knee, and base of thumb joints. The ankle joint can be fused or replaced.
  - **Arthroscopy lavage and debridement** – patients should only be referred if they have OA of the knee with a clear history of mechanical locking.

Self-assessment

A 68 year old female has been complaining of bilateral hip pain for the last 6 weeks. An X-ray is then performed (*Fig. 2.2.6*).

1. Describe any abnormalities you see in the X-ray.
2. What pharmacological agents would you begin with? If these don't work, what is your next plan of action?
3. She returns to your clinic some months later complaining that the medications are not working. What are the indications for surgical intervention and what procedure should be performed?

Answers to self-assessment questions are to be found in *Appendix A*.

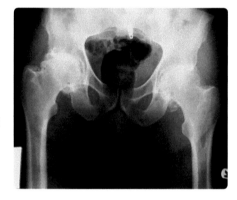

Fig. 2.2.6: X-ray of pelvis.

2.3 Septic arthritis

Septic arthritis is the **acute infection** (usually **bacterial**) of a **native** or **prosthetic joint**. Since septic arthritis can lead to **rapid joint destruction**, immediate accurate diagnosis and treatment are essential. Any joint can be affected, particularly the **lower limb joints**, most commonly the **hip** and **knee**.

Pathophysiology

- Septic arthritis usually occurs due to the spread of bacteria from another site to the joint:
  - The commonest route of spread is **haematogenous** (**respiratory** or **urinary tract infection (UTI)**).
  - Other routes include **local tissue infection** (**cellulitis** and **osteomyelitis**), **penetrating trauma** and **inoculation** (skin opportunistic pathogens may spread when there is a break in the skin).
- Release of **cytokines** leads to hydrolysis of **proteoglycans** and **collagen**, **cartilage destruction**, and eventually **bone loss** (if left untreated).
- **Bacteria** are the most common causative pathogens (*Fig. 2.3.1*). **Viruses** and **fungi** rarely cause septic arthritis.

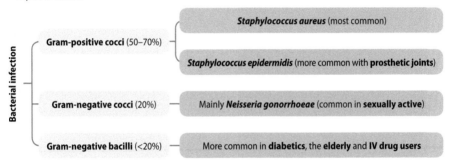

Fig. 2.3.1: Causative bacteria of septic arthritis.

Epidemiology and risk factors

- The estimated incidence of septic arthritis in the UK is 2–10 cases per 100 000 of the population.

Table 2.3.1: Risk factors for septic arthritis	
Prosthetic joint	• Incidence is 10 × higher. Early infection is most likely due to *Staphylococcus aureus*, whereas delayed infection is due to coagulase-negative staphylococcus and Gram-negative aerobes.
Rheumatoid arthritis	• Incidence is 10 × higher.
Diabetes mellitus	• Diabetic patients have increased risk of infection.
Low socioeconomic status	• Poverty and malnutrition, and those abusing alcohol and drugs.
Age	• Extremes of age (<15 and >55).
Intravenous drug use	• Transfer of pathogenic organisms via haematogenous spread.
Osteomyelitis	• Osteomyelitis from penetrating injuries can spread to joint.
Intra-articular injection / aspiration	• Transfer of pathogenic skin organisms directly into joint.

Clinical features

- Usually **one joint** is affected. However, less commonly two or more joints may be affected at the same time due to the spread of bacteria.
- The **knee** is the most common site of infection (**>50%**), followed by the **hip** (more common in **children**), then the **shoulder**, **wrist**, **elbow** and **ankle**. Other joints are rarely affected.
- **Symptoms / signs include**:

  - Extremely painful, red (erythema), swollen joint (acute).
  - **Muscle spasm** resulting in **joint immobility**.
  - **Systemic features** – tachycardia, fever, rash, malaise and anorexia.
  - **Loosening of the implant** (chronic infection in prosthetic joint).
- The clinical picture may be partially masked in the **elderly**, **immunocompromised**, those with **RA** and **IV drug users**.

> **Rapid diagnosis:** Septic arthritis in children (Kocher criteria for a child with a painful hip)
>
> - Non-weight-bearing on affected side
> - Raised ESR
> - Fever
> - Raised WCC
>
> Probability that child has septic arthritis:
> 4/4 = 99%, 3/4 = 93%, 2/4 = 40%, 1/4 = 3%

Diagnosis and investigations

Hx
- **Presenting complaint**: extreme pain, overlying skin is red, swollen joint and fever (60%). In most cases of septic arthritis there is a rapid onset of symptoms (<2 weeks) and only one joint is affected.
- **Past medical history** e.g. diabetes, RA and other risk factors (*Table 2.3.1*).
- **Social history**: low socioeconomic status and IV drug use.
- **Sexual history**: gonorrhoeal infection.

Ex
- **Look** → signs of erythema, swelling and obvious effusion.
- **Feel** → tenderness, warmth and effusion.
- **Move** → marked limitation of movements and inability to bear weight.
- Presence of systemic features (fever, malaise, rash and tachycardia).

Ix
- **Aspiration of the joint**: to obtain a sample of synovial fluid. Synovial fluid is sent for immediate Gram stain, WCC, culture and polarized light microscopy (to rule out gout / CPPD). May show presence of microorganisms; WCC is often raised. Subsequent culture reveals organism type and sensitivities to antibiotic therapy.
- **Blood culture**: presence of microorganisms; reveals organism type and sensitivities to antibiotic therapy.
- **Blood test**: ↑ESR, WCC and CRP. Electrolyte and liver function tests can be performed to indicate whether there is systemic sepsis.
- **X-ray**: usually normal but may reveal any underlying joint disease at presentation, e.g. RA.
- **Ultrasound**: may show presence of effusion to guide aspiration.

DDx		
	• Gout	• Flare-up of RA
	• Pseudogout	• Transient non-specific synovitis (hip)
	• Acute exacerbation of OA	• Reactive arthritis
	• Bursitis	• Haemarthrosis

Management

Antibiotics

- **Empirical antibiotics** (initially **IV**) whilst waiting for synovial fluid joint analysis (refer to local guidelines and consult microbiologist).
- The choice of empirical therapy depends on the most likely causative organism:
  - **Flucloxacillin** (0.5–1 g/6 hours IV for 4–6 weeks) for *Staphylococcus aureus* and **vancomycin** for **MRSA**.
  - If **penicillin-allergic** then **IV clindamycin** should be given (0.6–2.7 g daily in 2–4 divided doses for 4–6 weeks).
  - **Cefotaxime** (1 g every 12 hours IV for 4–6 weeks) for **gonococcal** or **Gram-negative bacteria**.
- Other antibiotics may be indicated and added, depending on the results of culture and sensitivity testing.
- Antibiotic therapy should be continued for at least **6 weeks**.

Non-pharmacological management

- **Orthopaedic review** for the consideration of **arthrocentesis**, **lavage** and **debridement**, particularly if **prosthetic joint** is affected.
- **Joint immobilization** followed by **physiotherapy**.
- **Regular review** and **examination** of the affected joint as well as follow-up blood tests for inflammatory markers.

Self-assessment

A 9 year old boy presents with an acute red, swollen hip and is unable to walk. You suspect that he has septic arthritis.

1. What findings would you expect on examination?
2. An aspiration of the joint is performed to obtain a sample of synovial fluid. What tests should be performed on the sample?
3. What is the most likely causative organism for sepsis in this case?
4. What empirical antibiotic would you prescribe?
5. List some risk factors of septic arthritis.

Answers to self-assessment questions are to be found in *Appendix A*.

Introduction to spondyloarthropathies

- Spondyloarthropathies are a group of inflammatory arthropathies which include the following conditions ('**PEAR**'):
  - **P**soriatic arthritis (*Sec. 2.4*)
  - **E**nteropathic spondyloarthropathies – associated with inflammatory bowel disease and GI bypass surgery (this condition is not discussed any further in this book)
  - **A**nkylosing spondylitis (*Sec. 2.5*)
  - **R**eactive arthritis (*Sec. 2.6*)
- The spondyloarthropathies frequently overlap and have several clinical features in common:
  - **Rheumatoid factor negative** (seronegative)
  - **HLA-B27 association** – HLA-B27-positive individuals have a 20-fold increased risk of developing a spondyloarthropathy
  - **Axial arthritis** – arthritis of the spine and sacroiliac joints
  - **Asymmetrical large joint oligoarthritis** (<5 joints) or **monoarthritis**
  - **Enthesitis** – inflammation of the site of tendon or ligament insertion e.g. plantar fasciitis and Achilles tendinitis
  - **Dactylitis** ('sausage digit') – inflammation of the entire digit as a result of soft tissue oedema, and tenosynovial and joint inflammation
  - **Extra-articular manifestations** – these differ from RA, e.g. inflammatory bowel disease (IBD) and iritis

---

The European Spondyloarthropathy Study Group criteria for spondyloarthropathy

Inflammatory spinal pain, or **synovitis** (asymmetric, predominantly in the lower extremities) and one or more of the following:
- **Family history**: first-degree or second-degree relative with **ankylosing spondylitis**, **psoriasis**, **acute iritis**, **reactive arthritis** or **IBD**
- Past or present **psoriasis**
- Past or present **IBD**
- Past or present pain alternating between the two buttocks
- Past or present spontaneous **enthesitis** on examination
- Episode of diarrhoea occurring within one month before onset of arthritis
- **Non-gonococcal urethritis** or **cervicitis** occurring within one month before onset of arthritis
- **Sacroiliitis** (meeting the criteria shown in *Fig. 2.5.2*)

2.4 Psoriatic arthritis

Psoriatic arthritis (PsA) is a **chronic inflammatory arthritis** and the most common type of **seronegative oligoarthritis**. PsA is unique compared to other **seronegative spondyloarthritides** in that the **small joints** of the **hand** are commonly affected. A variety of joint patterns are recognized in PsA, although these may overlap.

Pathophysiology

- The pathogenesis of PsA remains poorly understood.
- Like other autoimmune joint diseases, **genetically susceptible individuals** are exposed to an **environmental trigger** (**bacteria**, **stress**, or **entheseal-related peptide**) which may then activate the immune system.
- This results in **T-cell infiltration** and **chemokine / cytokine** release.
- The process is amplified by **angiogenesis** and **cellular infiltration** of involved tissues.
- **Human leucocyte antigen (HLA)** and other genes may determine the exact pattern of tissue involvement.

Epidemiology and risk factors

- The prevalence of PsA in the UK is approximately 2%.
- Men and women are equally affected.

Table 2.4.1: Risk factors for PsA	
Psoriasis	**Strongest risk factor**. Skin psoriasis may occur **before** (**70%**), **after** (**25%**), or at **same time as** (**5%**) joint symptoms.
Hereditary	Approx. **40%** of individuals with psoriasis or PsA have first-degree relatives with psoriasis or PsA. There is an association between **HLA-B27** and PsA.
Joint or tendon trauma	A small number of PsA patients may recall trauma prior to the onset of their arthritis.
HIV	The prevalence of PsA is higher in patients with HIV compared to the general population.
Age	More common in individuals aged **30–55** but can occur at any age.
Ethnicity	PsA is more common in **Caucasians** than Africans or Asians.

Clinical features

- A variety of PsA patterns of joint involvement are recognized (*Table 2.4.2*).

Table 2.4.2: Patterns of PsA – 'DR SAM'	
DIP joint disease (5–10%)	Predominantly **DIP** involvement (*Fig. 2.4.1*). Affects **men** more and is strongly associated with **onycholysis**.
Rheumatoid pattern (25%)	Presents very similarly to RA – **symmetrical small joint arthritis** particularly affecting **MCP, wrist** and **PIP joints**. Distinguishing features are **lack of nodules** and **negative** for **RF**.
Spondyloarthritis (20%)	May present with isolated **sacroiliitis**, **typical** or **atypical AS**.
Asymmetrical oligoarthritis (50%)	**Large joint inflammatory arthritis** often with **ankle, knee, wrist** or **shoulder** involvement.
Mutilans arthritis (1–5%)	Most **rare** but **severe** form. **Osteolysis** results in **destruction** of the **small joints** of the **digits** with **shortening** (*Fig. 2.4.2*).

- **General symptoms and signs**:
  - **Joint pain** and **stiffness** – inflammatory joint pain is characterized by prolonged morning stiffness (>30 mins), improvement with use, and recurrence with prolonged rest.
  - **Dactylitis** or 'sausage digits' (*Fig. 2.4.3*).
  - **Enthesitis** – pain, stiffness and tenderness of insertions into bone e.g. the Achilles tendon (*Fig. 2.4.4*).
  - Extra-articular features – **psoriatic skin rash** (*Fig. 2.4.5*), **nail changes** (pitting, onycholysis and hyperkeratosis) and **uveitis**.

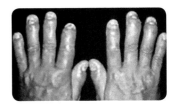

Fig. 2.4.1: DIP involvement in PsA – highly characteristic.

Rapid diagnosis: CASPAR criteria for PsA

Established inflammatory articular disease and ≥3 points is diagnostic of PsA:
A. **Current psoriasis** = 2 points
B. **History of psoriasis** (in the absence of A) = 1
C. **Family history of psoriasis** (in the absence of A or B) = 1
D. **Dactylitis** = 1
E. **Juxta-articular new bone formation** = 1
F. **RF negative** = 1
G. **Nail dystrophy** = 1

Fig. 2.4.2: Hands showing psoriatic arthritis mutilans.

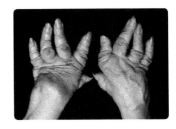

Fig. 2.4.3: 'Sausage toes'.

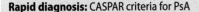

Diagnosis and investigations

Hx
- **Clinical presentation** (*see above*).
- **Family history** – psoriasis or psoriatic arthritis.
- **Past medical history** – psoriasis, history of scalp or nail problems, joint or tendon trauma and HIV.

Ex
- Recognition of the pattern of joint involvement is essential to the diagnosis of PsA (*Table 2.4.2*).
- **Swelling and tenderness** of individual joints (synovitis) during inspection and palpation.
- **'Sausage digits'**.
- **Skin**, **scalp** and **nail** involvement – patients may not know they have psoriasis!
- **Pain at site of tendon attachment** – commonly affected sites include **Achilles tendon**, **plantar fascia**, and **epicondyles**.
- **Spinal stiffness** with low back pain due to **sacroiliitis** (uncommon).

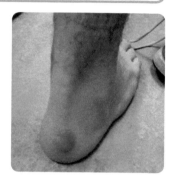
Fig. 2.4.4: Achilles tendon bursitis.

Ix
1. **X-rays**:
   - Soft tissue swelling may be the only radiographical finding seen in early disease.
   - Erosion in the DIP joint and periarticular new-bone formation; osteolysis and 'pencil-in-cup' deformity in advanced disease (*Fig. 2.4.6*).
2. **Blood tests**:
   - Normal or raised ESR and CRP (in active disease).
   - Immunology – RF, anti-CCP and antinuclear antibodies (ANA) negative.

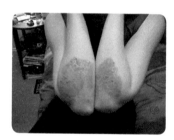
Fig. 2.4.5: Psoriatic skin rash.

DDx
- RA (symmetrical pattern)
- Erosive OA
- Gout (monoarthritic, large joint, especially knee)
- Reactive arthritis
- Sarcoid dactylitis

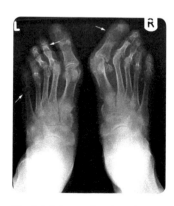
Fig. 2.4.6: Arrows show 'pencil-in-cup' deformity caused by underlying osteolysis.

Management

Table 2.4.3: Management of PsA	
NSAIDs	First-line for **pain relief** and **soft tissue inflammation**.
DMARDs	• First-line for those with **progressive peripheral joint disease** who require more aggressive treatment. • **Methotrexate** is usually the first-line DMARD. • Alternative DMARDs include **ciclosporin, sulfasalazine** and **leflunomide**. • The combination of methotrexate and ciclosporin is particularly effective. • An initial trial of a DMARD for PsA is **3 months**.
Intra-articular corticosteroid injections	• May be indicated if non-steroidal anti-inflammatory drugs (NSAIDs) alone are not sufficient for symptomatic relief. • Corticosteroid injection is given once and then reassessed.
Anti-TNF-α therapy	• Highly effective for **severe skin** and **joint disease**. • There is no preferred TNF-α inhibitor – **etanercept, adalimumab, infliximab** or **golimumab** can be used.
Physiotherapy	Helps improve range of motion and pain, as well as muscle strengthening of joints with associated periarticular muscle atrophy.

Self-assessment

A 52 year old male with a past medical history of psoriasis complains of symmetrical pain and swelling in both of his hands. You suspect psoriatic arthritis.

1. Apart than psoriatic skin rash, what are some of the other extra-articular features of psoriatic arthritis?
2. What clinical features and blood tests help to distinguish between rheumatoid arthritis and psoriatic arthritis?
3. An X-ray is later performed. What abnormalities might you see?
4. Name two pharmacological agents for pain relief in psoriatic arthritis.
5. Name the first-line pharmacological agent to prevent disease progression and its side-effects.

Answers to self-assessment questions are to be found in *Appendix A*.

2.5 Ankylosing spondylitis

Ankylosing spondylitis (AS) is the most common of the **seronegative spondyloarthropathies (SpA)**. It is a **chronic inflammatory** disorder of the **sacroiliac joints** and **spine**. Other clinical features include **peripheral arthritis**, **enthesitis**, and **extra-articular organ** involvement.

Pathophysiology

- Both **genetic** and **environmental** factors interplay in the pathogenesis of AS.
- **HLA-B27** is the most common predisposing gene in AS.
- The disease is first characterized by **inflammation** of the **sacroiliac (SI) joints**.
- SI joint involvement is followed by involvement of several structures including the **intervertebral discs**, **zygapophyseal**, **costovertebral** and the **costotransverse joints**, as well as the **paravertebral ligaments**.
- Early lesions include **subchondral granulation tissue** which erodes the joint and is replaced gradually by **fibrocartilage** and then ossification. This occurs in **ligamentous** and **capsular** attachment sites to bone (**enthesitis**).
- In the later stage, the outer layer of the **annulus fibrosis** starts to **calcify**, creating a bony bridge between the **vertebral bodies (syndesmophytes)**.
- These may then fuse with the vertebral body above, causing **ankylosis** (*Fig. 2.5.1*).

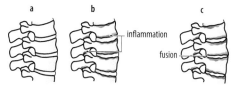

Fig. 2.5.1: **(a)** normal spine, **(b)** early AS, **(c)** advanced AS.

Epidemiology and risk factors

- AS is the most common seronegative SpA with a prevalence of 150 per 100 000 in the UK.
- A significant number of patients with mild symptoms remain undiagnosed.

Table 2.5.1: Risk factors for ankylosing spondylitis	
Genetics	• 90% of AS patients carry the **HLA-B27 gene**.
Gender	• Affects men more than women **(3:1)**.
Age	• Peaks at ages **17–35**.

Clinical features

- **Dull back pain** (radiating from the SI joints to the hips / buttocks) and **stiffness** >6 months. These symptoms are worse at night and in the early morning and are relieved by exercise and worsened by rest.
- **Reduced motion** in the **lumbar spine**, and **cervical spine movements** can be globally reduced.

Box 2.5.1: Extra-articular features of AS ('The A factor')

- **A**tlanto-axial subluxation
- **A**nterior uveitis
- **A**pical lung fibrosis
- **A**ortic incompetence
- **A**V (atrioventricular) node block
- **A**chilles tendinitis
- **A**myloidosis (a rare and late complication)

- Loss of **lumbar lordosis**.
- **Reduced chest expansion** due to progressive loss of spinal movements.
- **Thoracic kyphosis** and **neck hyperextension** ('**question mark posture**') – uncommon and occurs with progressive disease.
- **Peripheral synovitis** (approx. 30%). Typically asymmetrical oligoarthritis, most commonly affecting the hip and knee.
- **Extra-articular features** (*Box 2.5.1*).

OSCE tips: Schober's test

- The modified Schober's test examines flexion of the spine.
- An inferior mark at the level of **posterior superior iliac spines** is drawn and a **10 cm** segment above this point is marked on the patient's back.
- The increase in distance on maximal forward spinal flexion with **locked knees** is measured.
- The measured distance should increase from 10 cm to at least **13.5–15 cm** in healthy adults.

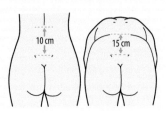

Diagnosis and investigations

- Based on the **modified New York (NY) criteria**, a definite diagnosis of AS requires the presence of radiological criteria and at least one clinical criterion (history and examination).

> **Hx** History of **back pain** and **stiffness** for longer than **3 months** which improves with exercise but is not relieved by rest.

> **Ex**
> - **Limitation of motion** of the **lumbar spine** in both **sagittal** and **frontal planes** (see *OSCE tips*).
> - **Limitation of chest expansion** to 1 inch or less.

> **Ix**
> - **X-ray** (modified NY radiological criterion): **Sacroiliitis grade ≥2 bilaterally** or **grade 3** or **4 unilaterally** (See *Fig. 2.5.2* for sacroiliitis grading).
> - Other radiographic features include:
>   - **Early**: Bone erosions, widening of the SI joints and vertebral bodies appear square with shiny corners (Romanus lesions).
>   - **Later**: Ossification of longitudinal ligaments of the spine (syndesmophytes) giving it a 'bamboo spine' appearance (*Fig. 2.5.3*).
> - **MRI scanning**: Although not included in the modified NY criteria, it is very useful for identifying early sacroiliitis and early inflammatory changes affecting the spine and therefore it can pick up AS at the early stages of the disease.
> - **Blood tests**: FBC normal, ↑CRP and ESR (active disease), RF and ANA negative, HLA-B27 (this has little role in diagnosis, but may indicate a predisposition to AS in the appropriate clinical context).
> - **Ultrasound scanning**: can help in diagnosing enthesitis.

DDx
- Mechanical back pain
- Other seronegative SpAs
- Degenerative lumbar or cervical spondylosis
- Trauma
- Infection
- Neoplasm

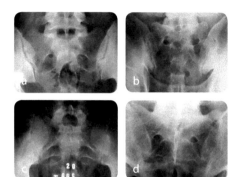

Fig. 2.5.2: Grading of sacroiliitis: **(a)** grade 0, normal; **(b)** grade I–II, mild sclerosis; **(c)** grade III, widening of joint space; **(d)** grade IV, bilateral ankylosis.

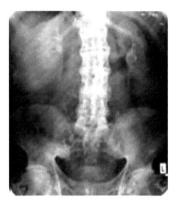

Fig. 2.5.3: X-ray of 'bamboo spine' in AS.

Management

- Early diagnosis and patient education are essential for effective AS management (*Table 2.5.2*).

Table 2.5.2: Management of AS based on Assessments in Ankylosing Spondylitis International Society (ASAS) / European League against Rheumatism (EULAR) recommendations

Exercise and physiotherapy	Intense exercises or activities such as badminton and swimming to strengthen muscle and provide better stability.
NSAIDs	First-line therapy for AS patients with pain and stiffness. Relieves symptoms and may slow radiographic progression. Examples – ibuprofen and naproxen.
Other analgesics	Offered when NSAIDs are insufficient or contraindicated. Examples – codeine and paracetamol.
Local corticosteroids	Temporarily relieve pain that does not respond well to NSAIDs.
Anti-TNF-α therapy	Given to patients with persistently high disease activity or if NSAIDs fail. Examples – adalimumab, etanercept and golimumab.
Surgery	Hip replacements are offered to patients with advanced hip involvement who suffer from refractory pain and disability.

- An instrument called the **Bath Ankylosing Spondylitis Disease Activity Index (BASDAI)** has been formulated for measuring the disease activity of AS by asking 6 questions related to 5 major symptoms of AS: **fatigue**, **spinal pain**, **arthralgia**, **enthesitis** and **morning stiffness**.

Self-assessment

A 22 year old male presents with low back pain and stiffness that has persisted for more than 3 months. His back symptoms are worse when he awakes in the morning, and the stiffness lasts more than 1 hour. There is no history of obvious injury.

1. What condition do you think this man has and why?
2. What special test would you perform on clinical examination? Describe how this is performed.
3. Which gene is strongly linked to the likely cause of his presentation?
4. What abnormalities might you see if an X-ray is performed on this man's lower back?
5. Outline a management plan for this patient.

Answers to self-assessment questions are to be found in *Appendix A*.

2.6 Reactive arthritis

Reactive arthritis is an **acute aseptic arthritis** that develops in response to an extra-articular infection, typically originating from the **gastrointestinal (GI)** or **genitourinary (GU) tract**. It is a **seronegative spondyloarthropathy** classically presenting with **asymmetrical oligoarthritis**, usually in the **lower limbs**.

Pathophysiology

- Reactive arthritis is thought to be caused by an **infectious trigger**, usually a **bacterial GI** or **GU infection** (*Fig. 2.6.1*) in **genetically susceptible individuals**.

- This leads to **immune activation** and **cross-reactivity** with **self-antigens** causing **acute inflammation** in the affected joint and other tissues approximately **2–6 weeks** after the initial infection.

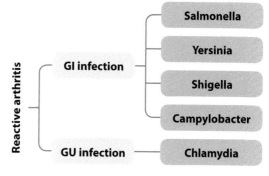

Fig. 2.6.1: The key GI and GU bacteria implicated in reactive arthritis.

- As well as inflammation of joints, inflammation of the **entheses, axial skeleton, skin, mucous membranes, GI tract** and **eyes** may also occur.

- **HLA-B27** is positive in most patients and it is not only a strong risk factor of reactive arthritis, but it may also predict the severity and chronicity of the disease.

Epidemiology and risk factors

- The estimated incidence of reactive arthritis in the UK is approximately 30–40 cases per 100 000 of the population.

Table 2.6.1: Risk factors for reactive arthritis

GI/GU infection	Reactive arthritis occurs after exposure to certain GI or GU infections.
Gender	There is a **9:1 male:female** incidence ratio of **Chlamydia-induced reactive arthritis** and **1:1** for **post-dysentery reactive arthritis**.
HLA-B27	HLA-B27 is positive in approximately **75%** of reactive arthritis patients.
Age	Most patients with reactive arthritis are **aged 20–40**.
Ethnicity	Reactive arthritis is more common in **Caucasians**.

Clinical features

- **Arthritis** – acute, asymmetrical large joint arthritis (often lower limbs), occurring 2–6 weeks after the initial infection (most often acute, and may be accompanied by malaise, fatigue and fever).
- Other features:
  - **Enthesitis** – plantar fasciitis and Achilles tendinitis.
  - **Conjunctivitis** (usually bilateral and painful) and **anterior uveitis** (usually unilateral).

- **Dactylitis** – may occur at one or more toes.
- **Urethritis** and **circinate balanitis** (ulcers and vesicles surrounding the glans penis).
- **Lower back pain** due to sacroiliitis and spondylitis.
- **Mouth ulcers**.
- **Nail dystrophy** and **keratoderma blennorrhagica** (*Fig. 2.6.2*).
- **Reiter's syndrome** – triad of **reactive arthritis**, **conjunctivitis** and **urethritis**. Although rare, it follows a GU or GI infection. It can be easily remembered using the mnemonic 'can't see, can't wee and can't bend your knee'!

Diagnosis and investigations

Hx
- **Presenting complaints**: peripheral arthritis, axial arthritis (sacroiliitis), systemic features (fever, fatigue and weight loss) and enthesitis are all common.
- **History of GI or GU infection** prior to infection.
- **Family history** of reactive arthritis.
- Consider a **sexual health review**.

Ex
- **Examine the affected joint(s)**.
- **Eyes** – conjunctivitis and uveitis.
- **Mouth** – oral ulcers.
- **Lower back** – pain due to sacroiliitis.
- **Genitals** – urethritis and circinate balanitis.
- **Foot** – plantar fasciitis, Achilles tendinitis, keratoderma blennorrhagica, 'sausage toes' and nail dystrophy.
- **Systemic features** – malaise, fatigue and fever.

Working downwards anatomically

Ix
- **Blood tests**: raised CRP, ESR, leucocytosis and thrombocytosis (acute phase), ANA, RF and anti-CCP are negative, HLA-B27 positive in 75%.
- **X-ray**: normal in early stages. Marginal erosions, plantar spurs, sacroiliitis and asymmetrical syndesmophytes may occur in chronic cases.
- **Joint aspiration**: to rule out crystal or septic arthritis. Synovial fluid is usually sterile and cloudy with high WCC.
- **Stool, throat or urine culture**: identify causative organism.
- **Serology**: for Chlamydia.
- **MRI**: asymmetrical sacroiliitis and enthesitis (chronic stage).

DDx	
	• Other seronegative spondyloarthropathies
	• Gonococcal arthritis
	• Gout
	• Inflammatory bowel disease
	• RA
	• Septic arthritis

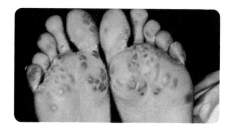

Fig. 2.6.2: Keratoderma blennorrhagica of the soles.

OSCE tips: Specific questions to ask someone with suspected reactive arthritis

- **Presenting complaint is usually asymmetrical joint pain**: Is it warm? Red? Sudden onset? Occurred after a bowel or urine infection? If so, how many days / weeks after?
- **Other complaints** (head to toe): Eye infection? Mouth ulcers? Back pain? Urine infection? Rash on penis? Pain or rash on soles of feet? Swollen toes? Fatigue? Fever?
- **Past medical history**: Recent stomach bug or urine infection?
- **Family history**: Has anyone in your family suffered from anything similar?
- **Sexual history**: Unprotected sex? New partner?

Management

Table 2.6.2: Management of reactive arthritis

Non-pharmacological	**Rest** and **splint** affected joint (acutely). Consider **physiotherapy**.
NSAIDs	For **pain relief** and **soft tissue inflammation**.
Corticosteroids	**Intra-articular**, for instance **sacroiliac joints** can be injected. A short course of **oral corticosteroids** can be considered for patients who are unresponsive to NSAIDs or who develop adverse effects. **Topical corticosteroids** can be used to treat skin involvement.
DMARDs	Particularly **methotrexate** and **sulfasalazine** have been shown to be beneficial for some patients; indicated for **persistent** or **refractory disease**.
Antibiotics	**Tetracyclines** may be useful for **urethritis** caused by **Chlamydia**.
Anti-TNF-α therapy	In more aggressive cases, or when reactive arthritis evolves towards AS, anti-TNF-α therapy may represent an effective choice.

Self-assessment

A 21 year old male presents with a 2 week history of an acute painful, hot, and swollen left knee, and low back pain with bilateral buttock pain. Further review of symptoms indicates the patient was treated for a Chlamydia infection after he developed dysuria approximately 2 months ago. You suspect reactive arthritis.

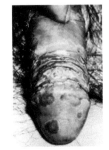

1. What risk factors predispose this patient to reactive arthritis?
2. On examination, why would you look at the soles of the feet?
3. What is the name of the reactive arthritis manifestation shown in *Fig. 2.6.3?*
4. What blood tests would you perform and what do you expect to find?
5. How would you manage this patient acutely?

Answers to self-assessment questions are to be found in *Appendix A*.

Fig. 2.6.3: Reactive arthritis manifestation.

2.7 Gout

Gout is an **inflammatory arthritis** which progresses from asymptomatic **hyperuricaemia** (elevated circulating **uric acid levels**). It is caused by deposition of **urate crystals** in the **synovial fluid** of **joints**, **bone** and other tissues.

Pathophysiology

- There is an association between gouty arthropathy and **hyperuricaemia** which is **often asymptomatic** for up to **20 years** before the initial attack (*Fig. 2.7.1*).

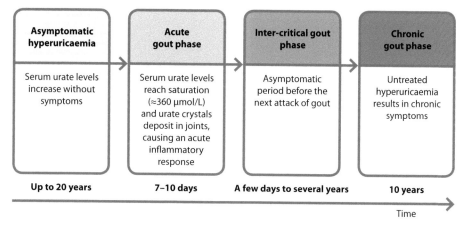

Fig. 2.7.1: Time scale of gout development.

- The build-up of **urate crystal** (a purine product) can be caused by **impaired renal excretion**, **overproduction of uric acid** and / or by **overconsumption of purine-rich foods** that are metabolized to **urate**.

Epidemiology and risk factors

- The **prevalence** of gout in the **UK** is approximately **1.4%** and is **increasing** (more common in countries such as the USA) because of obesity and dietary factors.
- The annual **incidence** of **acute attacks of gout** in the **UK** is around **12 cases per 10 000**.

Table 2.7.1: Risk factors for gout	
Hyperuricaemia	• The **most important risk factor** for gout (however, a high level does not confirm gout).
Male sex	• Approximately **4:1** male:female ratio.
Diet	• **Meat** (especially red meat) and **seafood** (especially shellfish).
Alcohol	• Alcohol is metabolized to **ketones** that compete with urate for renal excretion; alcohol also ↑ risk of gout via **dehydration**.
Drugs	• **Diuretics** (thiazide and loop), **aspirin**, **ciclosporin** and **laxatives**.
Chronic renal failure	• Inability to excrete urate.
Other risk factors	• **Obesity, hypertension, family history**, **age, coronary heart disease** and **diabetes mellitus**.

Clinical features

Most commonly affects the **first metatarso-phalangeal joint (MTP)** – gout here is also known as **podagra** (*Fig. 2.7.2a*). Other common sites include **small joints** of the **foot (mid-tarsal)** and **hand**, **the ankle**, **knee** and **elbow**.

- A **single peripheral joint** which becomes **excruciatingly painful** (often **nocturnal**), **red**, **hot** and **swollen** suggests <u>**acute gout**</u>.
- **Polyarthritis**, **tophi** (nodular subcutaneous deposition of uric acid crystals, see *Fig. 2.7.2b* and *c*), **fever and malaise** (uncommon) suggest <u>**chronic gout**</u> (**uric acid kidney stones** may also develop).

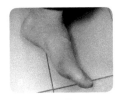

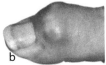

b

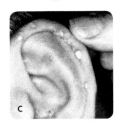

c

OSCE tips: Key questions to ask patients with suspected gout

- First time? Timing of onset and duration? Is it painful when socks are worn? Night attacks – painful with bed covers?
- Family history of gout / other arthritic conditions?
- Do you suffer from diabetes, hypertension or kidney problems? Do you take 'water pills'?
- Have you had any recent tests that included the injection of dye?
- Have you ever been told your serum urate levels are high?
- Diet habits and alcohol intake?

Fig. 2.7.2: **(a)** Gout of the big toe (podagra). Tophi affecting **(b)** DIP and **(c)** helix of the ear.

Diagnosis and investigations

Hx
- Typically, abrupt development of **severe joint pain** that reaches its maximum within **6–12 hours** and may undergo **remission** within **2 weeks (acute gout)**.
- **Risk factors** including age, family history, use of medication, diet and alcohol.

Ex
- **90%** of **gout attacks** are **monoarthritic**, and the majority occur in the **first MTP**.
- **Swelling, erythema, shiny surface and tenderness of the affected joint**.
- **Tophi** → **hallmark of chronic gout**.

Ix
- **Joint aspiration and synovial fluid analysis** → definitive diagnosis demonstrated by the presence of negatively birefringent crystals under polarized light microscopy.
- **Serum urate measurement** → often elevated. Useful for monitoring the response to treatment.
- **Radiographs** – soft tissue swelling (early), possibly punched-out erosions (later).

DDx
- Septic arthritis
- Pseudogout
- Acute flare of osteoarthritis (most common condition that affects the 1st MTP)
- Cellulitis

Management

- Confirm the diagnosis of gout and exclude other conditions, especially septic arthritis.
- The management of gout can be principally divided into prevention and treatment of acute attacks of gout (*Table 2.7.2*).

Table 2.7.2: Management and prevention of gout in accordance with NICE (2012)

Management of acute gout	
NSAIDs	Prescribe as soon as possible and continue until 48 hours after the gout has resolved. Use 'strong' NSAIDs, e.g. indomethacin (50 mg/8 hours), or naproxen (0.5–1 g daily). Co-prescribe a PPI in high-risk individuals.
Colchicine	If NSAIDs are contraindicated, not tolerated, or have been ineffective in previous attacks, prescribe oral colchicine (0.5 mg/6 hours).
Corticosteroids	If NSAIDs and colchicine are contraindicated, e.g. in renal impairment, consider a short course of oral systemic corticosteroids. Intra-articular corticosteroids are an option if no more than 2 joints are affected.
Paracetamol	With / without codeine, in addition to above drugs or alone, solely for pain relief.
Prevention of gout	
Lifestyle changes	↓ Body weight, ↓ excessive consumption of food rich in purines (meat and seafood), ↓ alcohol, take regular exercise and stop smoking.
Allopurinol	Start allopurinol 1–2 weeks after inflammation has settled and titrate the dose until serum uric acid (SUA) level <300 μmol/L. Co-prescribe a low-dose NSAID, or low-dose colchicine, for at least 1 month to prevent acute attacks of gout. Avoid stopping allopurinol in subsequent acute attacks once established on treatment.
Febuxostat	Consider as second-line therapy if allopurinol is contraindicated / not tolerated.

Self-assessment

A 55 year old obese male complains of a sudden onset painful, red and swollen big toe. A diagnosis of crystal arthritis is strongly suspected.

1. Which conditions would you consider in your differential diagnosis? Name the most important one and state why.

2. What are the typical clinical features of an attack of acute gout?

3. What risk factors predispose the patient to gout?

4. A joint aspiration is performed. How would you examine the aspirate and what results would you expect?

5. An X-ray (*Fig. 2.7.3*) is taken. What abnormalities does it show?

6. What are the main treatments for acute gout? What are the side-effects of these medications?

7. How can recurrent attacks of gout be prevented?

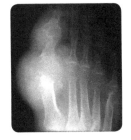

Fig. 2.7.3: X-ray of the foot.

Answers to self-assessment questions are to be found in *Appendix A*.

Calcium pyrophosphate disease

Calcium pyrophosphate disease (CPPD), often referred to as **pseudogout**, is caused by the deposition of **calcium pyrophosphate crystals** into the **joint space**. CPPD commonly coexists with **osteoarthritis** and is the most common cause of **chondrocalcinosis** (**calcification of cartilage** seen on X-ray).

Pathophysiology

- **Calcium pyrophosphate (CPP) crystals** form **extracellularly** when **inorganic pyrophosphate** reacts with **calcium**.
- The crystals first deposit in the joint **cartilage** (**fibrocartilage** and **hyaline cartilage**) which can result in **inflammation** and later damage to the cartilage and surrounding tissue.
- This deposition can result in **chondrocalcinosis**.

Epidemiology and risk factors

- The prevalence of **CPPD** is ~**7%** in the **UK**.
- Men and women are equally affected.

Clinical features

- May be **asymptomatic** but picked up on routine X-ray.
- Acute **tender**, **red**, **hot**, **swollen joint** suggests **acute CPPD** (also known as **pseudogout**).
- **Pain** and **stiffness** with long-term damage to joints (usually **knees**, **wrists**, **hips, and shoulders**) suggests **chronic CPPD**.

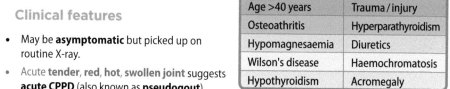

Table 2.8.1: Risk factors for CPPD

Age >40 years	Trauma / injury
Osteoathritis	Hyperparathyroidism
Hypomagnesaemia	Diuretics
Wilson's disease	Haemochromatosis
Hypothyroidism	Acromegaly

OSCE tips: Gout vs CPPD	
Gout	**CPPD**
Negatively birefringent crystals under polarized light microscopy	Positively birefringent crystals under polarized light microscopy
Deposition of monosodium urate crystals	Deposition of CPP crystals
Typically affects 1st MTP; ankle and mid-tarsal joints are also commonly affected	Typically affects larger joints, e.g. knee, wrist and ankle
More common in men	Equal sex distribution
Presentation is similar for both acute gout and acute CPPD, but there is usually a difference in joint distribution	
Acute management for both conditions is very similar (NSAIDs and colchicine); allopurinol has no role in the prevention of CPPD	

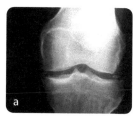

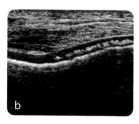

Fig. 2.8.1: **(a)** Plain X-ray showing CPP deposition in the fibrocartilage of the knee (chondrocalcinosis). **(b)** Ultrasound of the knee showing similar deposition.

Diagnosis and investigations

Hx
- **Severe joint pain** and **swelling** that reaches its maximum within **6–24 weeks** is likely to be acute crystal inflammation, though this is not specific for acute CPP crystal arthritis.
- **Risk factors** (*Table 2.8.1*).

Ex
- **Large joints** affected, e.g. knee.
- **Tenderness** and **erythema**.
- **Signs** of the **underlying cause**, e.g. **osteoarthritis**.

Ix
- **Blood tests**: ↑WCC, ↑ESR, ↑CRP (acute attack).
- **Joint X-rays**: chondrocalcinosis (*Fig. 2.8.1a*) and changes of OA.
- **Ultrasound**: (*Fig. 2.8.1b*).
- **Aspiration of the joint and synovial fluid analysis**: ↑WCC. Positive birefringent rhomboid-shaped crystals (i.e. CPP crystals) under polarized light microscopy. The joint fluid may appear purulent in nature.

DDx
- Septic arthritis
- Gout
- Osteoarthritis (chronic CPPD)
- Cellulitis

Management

- Any underlying causes need to be managed appropriately.
- Optimal treatment requires both non-pharmacological and pharmacological treatments.
  - **Non-pharmacological management** – initial rest followed by gradual mobilization of the joint. **Ice packs** may have a role in the short term for symptom relief.
  - **Pharmacological management** – **NSAIDs**, **colchicine**, intra-articular injection of long-acting **corticosteroids**.

Vasculitis

Vasculitides (singular, vasculitis) are a heterogeneous group of diseases that are categorized by inflammation of blood vessels, leading to compromise of the vascular lumen and ischaemia. The commonest form of vasculitis is **giant cell arteritis** (**GCA**; see *Sec. 2.10*). Other less common vasculitides include **Takayasu's arteritis**, **polyarteritis nodosa (PAN)**, **Wegener's granulomatosis (WG)**, **Churg–Strauss syndrome (CSS)** and **Henoch–Schönlein purpura (HSP)**.

Pathophysiology

Vasculitides can affect small, medium or large vessels (mainly arterial vessels).

Disease aetiology can be classified into either:

- **Primary** (idiopathic, which are autoimmune disorders and account for 45–55% of vasculitides) (*Fig. 2.9.1*).
- **Secondary**, mainly due to:
  - **infection** (15–20%) such as hepatitis B and C, tuberculosis (TB) and syphilis
  - **connective tissue disease** (15–20%) such as SLE, mixed connective tissue disease (MCTD) and RA
  - **drugs** (10–15%) e.g. hydralazine, propylthiouracil, sulphonamides, beta-lactams and quinolones

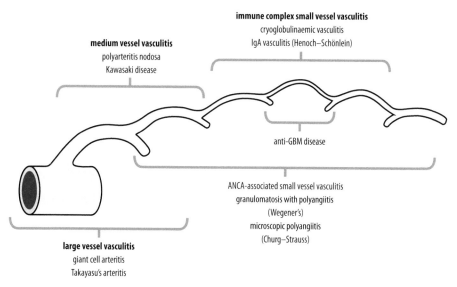

Fig. 2.9.1: Vasculitis classification. International Chapel Hill Consensus Conference Nomenclature of Vasculitides (CHCC 2012).

Table 2.9.1: Classification of vasculitis

Category	Condition	Definition
Large arteries	**Giant cell arteritis (GCA)**	Discussed in *Section 2.10*.
	Takayasu's arteritis	Granulomatous inflammation of the large arteries supplying the arm, head, neck and heart, leading to aortic arch syndrome. Occurs mainly in young women.
Medium arteries	**Polyarteritis nodosa (PAN)**	PAN is **necrotizing arteritis** without **glomerulonephritis** and is not associated with ANCA. This can lead to aneurysm, thrombosis and infarction.
Small arteries (c-ANCA and/or p-ANCA +ve)	**Granulomatosis with polyangiitis (Wegener's)**	A necrotizing vasculitis which is usually associated with granulomatous inflammation of the **respiratory tract** and glomerulonephritis.
Small arteries (p-ANCA +ve)	**Churg–Strauss syndrome (CSS)**	Eosinophil-rich and necrotizing granulomatous inflammation associated with asthma and eosinophilia.
	Microscopic polyangiitis (MPA)	Necrotizing vasculitis causing glomerulonephritis.
Small arteries (ANCA –ve)	Anti-glomerular basement membrane (GBM) disease	Vasculitis affecting glomerular capillaries, pulmonary capillaries, or both, with deposition of anti-basement membrane autoantibodies.
Immune complex small vessel vasculitis	**Henoch–Schönlein purpura (HSP)**	IgA dominant immune deposition. Usually affects the skin and GI tract and frequently causes arthritis.
Variable vessel vasculitis	Behçet's syndrome	Vasculitis that can affect arteries or veins, although mainly venules. Almost any organ can be affected. Common in those of Turkish descent, and very rare in the UK.

Epidemiology and risk factors

- Vasculitis is a rare condition.
- Epidemiology varies, depending on the gender, the subtype of vasculitis and the geographical location.

Table 2.9.2: Risk factors for vasculitis	
Other disorders	• RA and SLE can cause secondary vasculitis. • A history of **asthma and / or nasal allergies** is associated with CSS.
Age	• WG and CSS occur mainly in those aged >40. • HSP occurs mainly in children and young adults.
Gender	• Large vessel vasculitis is more common in women. • PAN affects men more than women.
Infection	• Syphilis, TB and hepatitis B and C are associated with secondary vasculitis.
Ethnicity	• Many forms of vasculitis are more common in Caucasian patients compared to other ethnicities. • Behçet's disease common in those of Turkish descent.
Geographical and environmental factors	• WG is more common amongst northern Europeans and commonly presents in winter following respiratory infection. • Microscopic polyangiitis is more common in southern Europe.

Clinical features

Takayasu's arteritis

- Usually presents with claudication of the arm.
- Loss of arm pulses, variation in blood pressure >10 mmHg between arms.

Polyarteritis nodosa (PAN)

- Presents with ischaemia or infarction within affected organs:
  - **GI tract** – **abdominal pain**, bleeding or perforation
  - **Heart** – angina or MI
  - **Kidneys** – hypertension and renal failure
  - **Peripheral nerves** – mononeuritis multiplex (due to inflammation of vessels supplying the nerve)
- Other presentations include weight loss, fever, raised diastolic blood pressure (>90 mmHg) and livedo reticularis (*Fig. 2.9.2*).
- PAN is common secondary to hepatitis B virus (HBV) infection.

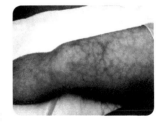

Fig. 2.9.2: Livedo reticularis on the anterior surface of the thigh.

Granulomatosis with polyangiitis, also known as Wegener's granulomatosis (WG)

A typical presentation involves the upper respiratory tract, lungs and kidneys:

- **Upper airway**
  - Nasal obstruction and crusting, with rhinorrhoea
  - Epistaxis, hyposmia (due to mucosal swelling) and epiphora (watering eye) due to involvement of the nasolacrimal duct and lacrimal sac

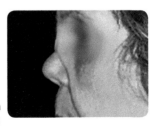

Fig. 2.9.3: Saddle nose deformity.

- Scleritis / episcleritis
- Sinusitis, nasal septal perforation and saddle nose deformity (*Fig. 2.9.3*)
- Recurrent otitis media (diminished hearing)
- Subglottic stenosis is classical feature in WG present with hoarseness of voice.
- **Pulmonary airway**
  - A common radiological feature is the presence of single or multiple **cavitary nodules** (*Fig. 2.9.4*) at cortical and sub-pleural sites
  - This can manifest as a persistent cough (usually unproductive), pyrexia, haemoptysis, dyspnoea and post-obstructive infection.
- **Kidneys**
  - Nephritic syndrome (haematuria, proteinuria, hypertension and uraemia).

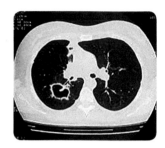

Fig. 2.9.4: Cavitary WG nodule in the right lung.

Other clinical features include skin rash (palpable purpura), conjunctival haemorrhages and scleritis.

The pathological hallmarks of WG are chronic granulomatous inflammation and vasculitis.

Churg–Strauss syndrome

- Classically presents with skin lesions (purpura or nodules) and mononeuritis multiplex with asthma.
- 50% have abdominal pain due to mesenteric arteritis.

Microscopic polyangiitis (MPA)

- Shares many similarities with WG. Classically presents with rapidly progressive glomerulonephritis and sometimes alveolar haemorrhage.
- Common symptoms include tiredness, loss of appetite, myalgia and arthralgia.

Anti-glomerular basement membrane (GBM) disease

- Usually presents as part of the classic Goodpasture's syndrome.
- Goodpasture's syndrome is defined by the triad of anti-GBM antibodies, glomerulonephritis and pulmonary haemorrhage.

Henoch–Schönlein purpura (HSP)

- Typically presents with palpable purpuric rash (small raised reddish / purple bumps; *Fig. 2.9.5*) over buttocks and lower leg.
- Abdominal pain and asymmetrical arthritis following upper respiratory tract infection.
- Glomerulonephritis occurs in 40% of patients.

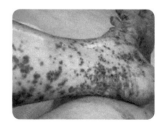

Fig. 2.9.5: Purpuric rash.

Behçet's disease

Behçet's disease is a systemic vasculitis of unknown cause. Typical presentation includes:

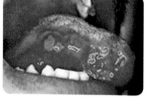

- Oral ulceration (*Fig. 2.9.6*)

- Genital ulceration

- Ocular involvement (anterior and posterior uveitis or retinal vascular lesions)

- Cutaneous lesions (including erythema nodosum or papulopustular rash)

Fig. 2.9.6: Oral ulceration.

- Arthritis (mono- or oligo-)

- GI features, including diarrhoea and anorexia

- Neurological features, including encephalitis, confusion or cranial nerve palsy.

Diagnosis and investigations

> **Hx**
> - Secondary vasculitis → any connective tissue disorders, recent infection and drug history.
> - Ask about asthma and recent blood transfusions (HBV).

> **Ex** **General examination**
> - **Skin**:
>   - Palpable purpura – HSP, WG, CSS
>   - Nodules, papules, ulcers, digital ischaemia – PAN
>   - Vesiculobullous (blisters) lesion – CSS, HSP
>   - Pallor – seen in any vasculitis
> - **Blood pressure**:
>   - Hypertension – PAN
> - **Oral cavity**:
>   - Strawberry tongue, lip cracking, congestion of oropharyngeal mucosa – Kawasaki syndrome
>   - Strawberry gums, gum ulceration – WG
>   - Oral ulcers – hallmark of Behçet's disease
> - **Other**:
>   - *Nose*: septal perforation, saddle nose deformity, mucosal ulceration – WG
>   - *Pulse*: unequal pulse between left and right sides – Takayasu's arteritis
>
> **Systematic examination**
> *Respiratory system*: asthma – CSS
> *CVS*: congestive heart failure – CSS
> *GI*: abdominal tenderness (mesenteric ischaemia) – PAN
> *MSK*: migratory polyarthritis – WG, CSS, MPA

Ix

Blood tests:

- **FBC**: normocytic anaemia; leucocytosis (e.g. eosonophilia), thrombocytosis (primary vasculitis); leucopenia or thrombocytopenia (secondary vasculitis)
- **Electrolytes**: hyperkalaemia in renal failure
- Raised **creatinine** in renal failure
- LFT abnormal in hepatitis B or C (may need to test for serology to confirm / rule out)

Immunology:

- Presence of c-ANCA and anti-proteinase 3 (anti-PR3) is very specific (>90%) for WG
- Presence of p-ANCA and anti-MPO is seen in MPA and CSS

Urine dipstick (glomerulonephritis)

Imaging:

- CXR (lung involvement) and echocardiogram (cardiac abnormalities)
- Angiograph: look for aneurysms, stenosis and post-stenotic dilatations in Takayasu's and PAN

Biopsy of the suspected vessel:

- Commonly taken from the site where vasculitis is suspected; e.g. temporal artery, nasal mucosa, sinuses and skin

Skin pathergy test:

- Performed when Behçet's syndrome suspected (very specific)
- Needleprick leads to papule formation within 48 hrs

DDx

- Primary vasculitis
- Secondary vasculitis
- Peripheral vascular disease, e.g. venous thromboembolism
- Antiphospholipid syndrome

Management

General principles:

- **Induce remission**; this can be achieved by **high-dose steroids** or **cyclophosphamide** (both orally and intravenously).
- Once remission is induced, the dose of steroid is **gradually reduced** and a **steroid-sparing agent** such as **methotrexate** or **azathioprine** is started.
- The patient is **maintained** on **low-dose steroids** and a steroid-sparing agent whilst being actively monitored.
- Additional therapies include angioplasty, plasma exchange and biological agents such as an IL-6 inhibitor.
- Supportive therapy such as analgesia and anti-inflammatory drugs are given when needed.

Self-assessment

A 35 year old woman presents with recurrent otitis media. She has a history of numerous episodes of epistaxis. On examination you notice that she has a prominent saddle nose, dark crusts in her nose and diminished hearing. Nasal mucosal biopsy shows granulomata and large areas of necrosis. Blood tests show positive c-ANCA.

1. What is the most likely diagnosis?
2. What other signs and symptoms may she have?
3. What is the pharmacological agent of choice for this condition?

Answers to self-assessment questions are to be found in *Appendix A*.

Giant cell arteritis

Giant cell arteritis (GCA) is the commonest form of vasculitis, typically affecting the **temporal artery**.

Pathophysiology

- GCA is an autoimmune disorder, where exposure to an unknown environmental trigger causes breakdown of immune tolerance, resulting in an autoimmune reaction against the arterial wall.
- GCA mainly affects the **extra-cranial branches** of the **carotid artery**, specifically the **temporal artery**. However, it can affect any branch of the aorta.
- The histopathological hallmark of GCA is the predominance of mononuclear infiltrates or granulomas, usually with **multinucleated giant cells**.
- Inflammatory cells stimulate the release of metalloproteases (MMPs) and reactive oxygen species (ROS) which damage the extracellular matrix of the blood vessel wall.

Epidemiology and risk factors

- GCA is the most common vasculitis in the UK, with approximately 13 000 new cases each year.

Table 2.10.1: Risk factors for primary vasculitis

Polymyalgia rheumatica	• 50% of patients with GCA have PMR.
Age	• GCA occurs almost exclusively in patients >50 years old.
Gender	• GCA is 3 × more common in females.
Ethnicity	• Mainly affects Caucasians.

Clinical features

- Abrupt-onset **headache**, usually unilateral in the temporal area.
- **Scalp pain**.
- Temporal artery **tenderness** and **swelling** (*Fig. 2.10.1*) with loss of pulsation.
- **Visual symptoms**, due to ophthalmic artery involvement, are a very serious complication of GCA. Specific symptoms of visual involvement should always be asked. These should not be missed and include:
  - **Amaurosis fugax** (transient loss of vision in one eye)
  - Blurring and diplopia
  - Partial or complete loss of vision
- **Jaw** and **tongue claudication**
- Systemic features of PMR commonly include: fever, fatigue, weight loss and muscle aching.

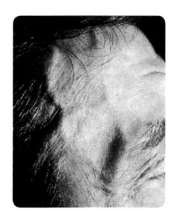

Fig. 2.10.1: Swollen temporal artery in GCA patient.

Diagnosis and investigations

Hx
- Ask about whether they have polymyalgia rheumatica (PMR) or PMR symptoms.
- Ask about visual symptoms (amaurosis fugax, diplopia, and partial or complete loss of vision).
- Patient might complain of jaw claudication ('Painful jaw when chewing?').
- Sudden onset of severe headache, often in the temporal or occipital region; worse at night.

Ex

Vascular:
- Scalp tenderness
- Tenderness of temporal artery and / or decreased temporal artery pulse
- Carotid bruits might be heard on auscultation
- Abdominal bruits or abnormal pulsatile aneurysmal swelling

Examination of the eye and vision:
- Ophthalmoscopic examination may reveal pale optic disc associated with severe loss of vision acuity
- Referral to ophthalmologist to perform slit-lamp examination may be required.

Ix

Blood tests:
- ↑ ESR ≥50 mm/hour.
- FBC → normocytic, normochromic anaemia, thrombocytosis.

Biopsy of the suspected vessel:
- Biopsy of the involved vessel may show a typical appearance of intermittent inflammation ('skip lesions'), or it may even be negative (20–30%).

Imaging:
- Ultrasound may reveal thickening of the affected blood vessel wall ('halo sign').

DDx
- Migraine
- Tension headache
- Trigeminal neuralgia

Rapid diagnosis box: The ACR classification criteria for GCA

1. **Age** at disease onset ≥50 years.
2. **New headache** (localized pain in the head).
3. **Temporal artery abnormality** (tenderness to palpation or decreased pulsation).
4. **Elevated ESR** (≥50 mm/hour).
5. **Abnormal artery biopsy** – mononuclear cell infiltration or granulomatous inflammation, usually with multinucleated giant cells).

For purposes of classification, a patient shall be said to have giant cell (temporal) arteritis if at least 3/5 criteria are present.

Management

- Immediate initiation of **high-dose glucocorticoid** treatment after clinical suspicion of GCA is raised.
- Visual loss occurs early in the course of disease and is irreversible.
- Early treatment with high-dose glucocorticoid is essential to prevent any further visual deterioration.

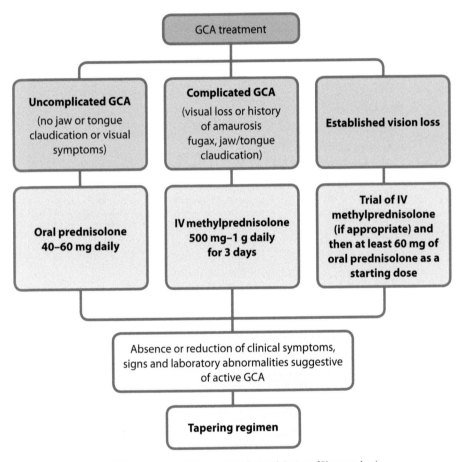

Fig. 2.10.2: Overview of GCA management (*Adapted from the British Society of Rheumatology*).

- Bone protection, such as a **bisphosphonate** and **calcium / vitamin D supplementation**, should be strongly considered.
- Tapering regimen: 40–60 mg prednisolone continued for 4 weeks. Then reduce dose by 10 mg every 2 weeks to 20 mg. Then by 2.5 mg every 2–4 weeks to 10 mg. Then by 1 mg every 1–2 months (provided there is no relapse).

Self-assessment

A 60 year old female presents with partial vision loss in her left eye. She complains of bitemporal headache for several weeks, along with pain and stiffness in the neck and shoulders. There are also signs of low grade fever, fatigue and weight loss. On physical examination, there is tenderness of the scalp over the temporal areas as well as thickening of the temporal arteries.

1. What is the most likely diagnosis?
2. What medication should be immediately administered?
3. Why does this patient have stiffness in the neck and shoulders?
4. What specific blood test would you request?
5. You request a temporal artery biopsy to confirm diagnosis and it comes back normal. Does this exclude your initial diagnosis?

Answers to self-assessment questions are to be found in *Appendix A*.

2.11 Polymyalgia rheumatica

Polymyalgia rheumatica (PMR) is an **inflammatory condition** that results in **muscle pain** and stiffness in the **shoulder** and **pelvic girdle**. **Giant cell arteritis (GCA)** is a more serious condition which usually coexists with PMR.

Pathophysiology

- Cause is unknown; genetic polymorphisms and environmental factors contribute to disease susceptibility.
- Association of HLA-DR4 has been reported in various population studies.
- **Inflammation is central to the pathogenesis of PMR**.

Epidemiology and risk factors

- The incidence of the disease in patients over 50 is around 100 per 100 000 in the UK.
- PMR is mainly seen in people of **north European** ancestry.

Table 2.11.1: Risk factors for PMR	
Age	• Almost exclusively present in patients **over the age of 50**, with peak incidence at age 65.
Gender	• Female:male, **3:1**.
Giant cell arteritis	• Approximately 40–60% of those with GCA have PMR.
Genetics	• Having siblings with PMR increases the risk.

Clinical features

- **Bilateral shoulder** (90%) or **thigh muscle aching pain persisting** for ≥1 month
- **Morning stiffness** lasting for >1 hour.
- Systemic features:
  - Loss of appetite
  - **Weight loss**
  - Low grade malaise
  - **Signs and symptoms of GCA**
  - Depression
- **It's important to exclude other conditions such as active infection, malignancy and GCA!**
- Main characteristic of PMR is the prompt **response to corticosteroids**.

Rapid diagnosis: British Society for Rheumatology guidelines

- **Age >50 years, duration >2 weeks**
- **Bilateral shoulder or pelvic girdle aching, or both**
- **Morning stiffness duration of >45 min**
- **Evidence of an acute-phase response, e.g. raised CRP**

Diagnosis and investigations

Hx
- Presence of risk factors e.g. age (>50 years).
- Acute onset shoulder / hip girdle pain and stiffness.
- Systemic features: low grade malaise, weight loss, depression.

Ex
- Normal muscle strength at initial presentation.
- There may be muscle tenderness proximally.
- **Temporal artery tenderness** suggests coexisting GCA.

Ix
Blood tests:
- Inflammatory markers:
  - **Raised ESR → >40 mm/hour**
  - Raised CRP
  - Urea and electrolytes → kidney function
- Serum protein electrophoresis → measures **paraprotein level to exclude multiple myeloma**.
- Thyroid function test → **exclusion of thyroid diseases**.
- Radiography → exclusion of non-erosive joint disease.
- Temporal artery biopsy → if GCA is clinically suspected.

DDx
- Polymyositis
- Metabolic bone e.g. osteomalacia
- Hypothyroidism
- Elderly onset of RA
- Fibromyalgia
- Possible underlying malignancy, e.g. multiple myeloma

Management

- Start with standardized daily dose of 15–20 mg **prednisolone. Clinical response of >70% in one week** is expected in PMR. Inflammatory markers should be normalized in 4 weeks.
- The dose of prednisolone is reduced slowly for 3–6 months to a low maintenance level which is sustained for a further 6–12 months then gradually reduced over the next 6 months, with the aim of stopping altogether.
- Due to long-term use of steroids, bone protective agent (e.g. **bisphosphonate**) and gastroprotective agent (e.g. **proton pump inhibitor (PPI)**) should be used.
- Most treatment can be discontinued after 18–24 months.
- Steroid-sparing agents, such as methotrexate and azathioprine, may also be used. Patients should be **monitored for the emergence of GCA**.
- If GCA occurs, then a higher initial prednisolone dose should be used (40–60 mg / day).

Self-assessment

A 56 year old female presents with a 4 week history of fatigue, weight loss, fevers, and bilateral pain and stiffness in the shoulder and hip girdles. She experiences difficulty getting out of bed in the morning due to stiffness, but these symptoms improve as the day progresses.

1. What is the most likely diagnosis? Give reasons for this.
2. What further questions would you like to ask to exclude other important differentials?
3. What investigations would you perform and why?
4. How should this patient be managed?

Answers to self-assessment questions are to be found in *Appendix A*.

Systemic lupus erythematosus

Systemic lupus erythematosus (SLE) is a **chronic multi-systemic autoimmune disease** of unknown cause that most commonly affects **women** during their **reproductive years**. Since it can affect any organ system, its presentation and course are highly variable. The disease is characterized by the presence of **antinuclear antibodies (ANA)**. There are other types of lupus (other than systemic), for instance **discoid lupus**, **drug-induced lupus** and overlap syndromes.

Pathophysiology

- Although the specific cause of SLE is unknown, multiple factors are associated with the development of the disease, including **genetic** and **environmental factors** such as **oxidative stress**, **infections**, **UV light exposure** and **drugs (drug-induced lupus)**.
- Many **innate** and **acquired** immune disturbances occur in SLE, which eventually results in the development of **autoantibodies** and **autoreactive T-cells** (*Fig. 2.12.1*).
- Defective clearance of **apoptotic cells** and **immune complexes** also contributes to the pathogenesis, and activation of the **complement system** plays a major role in tissue damage.
- **Antiphospholipid antibodies** are a specific family of autoantibodies directed against **anionic phospholipids** located in cell membranes (**antiphospholipid syndrome**, see *Box 2.12.2*).

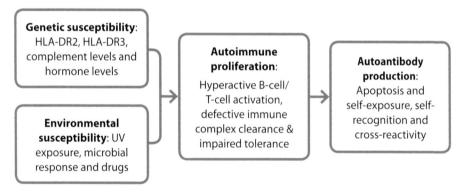

Fig. 2.12.1: Summary of pathogenesis of SLE.

Epidemiology and risk factors

- The prevalence of SLE is approximately 28 cases per 100 000 in the UK.
- The incidence of SLE is approximately 4 cases per 100 000 in the UK.

Table 2.12.1: Risk factors for SLE	
Female sex	• The female to male ratio is approximately **10:1**.
Age	• The incidence increases in women of **childbearing age (15–45)**.
Ethnicity	• More common in **Afro-Caribbeans** and **Asians**.
Drugs	• **Minocycline, isoniazid, terbinafine, phenytoin, carbamezapine** and **sulfasalazine** can cause drug-induced lupus.
Sun exposure	• May be an important environmental trigger of SLE.
Family history	• Genetic factors include **HLA, complement, Fc gamma receptor, cytotoxic T-lymphocyte antigen-4** and **cytokine genes**.
Tobacco smoking	• Smoking is linked not only to the development of SLE but also to the prognosis of the disease.

Clinical features

- SLE is a remitting and relapsing illness, typically presenting with non-specific constitutional symptoms of **malaise**, **fatigue**, **myalgia** and **fever**.
- See *Box 2.12.1* for specific features.
- Other features include **lymphadenopathy**, **weight loss**, **alopecia**, **nail-fold infarcts**, **non-infective endocarditis**, **Raynaud's**, **migraine**, **stroke**, and **retinal exudates**.

Box 2.12.1: The American College of Rheumatology revised criteria

Any four or more of the eleven criteria are required to classify a patient as having SLE. It can easily be memorized using the mnemonic 'SOAP BRAIN MD':

1. **S**erositis (one of the following):
   - Pleuritis: convincing history of pleuritic pain, pleural rubs on auscultation, or evidence of pleural effusion.
   - Pericarditis: documented by ECG, pericardial rub, or evidence of pericardial effusion.
2. **O**ral ulcers: oral or nasopharyngeal ulceration, usually painless, observed by physician.
3. **A**rthritis: non-erosive arthritis involving ≥2 peripheral joints, characterized by tenderness, swelling, or effusion.
4. **P**hotosensitivity: skin rash as a result of unusual reaction to sunlight, by patient history or physician observation.
5. **B**lood disorders (one of the following):
   - Haemolytic anaemia: with reticulocytes
   - Leucopenia: $<4 \times 10^9$/L on ≥2 occasions
   - Lymphopenia: $<1.5 \times 10^9$/L on ≥2 occasions
   - Thrombocytopenia: $<100\,000 \times 10^9$/L in the absence of offending drugs
6. **R**enal disorder: persistent proteinuria >0.5 g/day or >3+ if quantification not performed. Cellular casts: may be red cell, haemoglobin, granular, tubular or mixed.
7. **A**NA positive: an abnormal titre of ANA by immunofluorescence or an equivalent assay at any point in time and in the absence of drugs known to be associated with drug-induced lupus syndrome. Positive in >95%.

Box 2.12.1: The American College of Rheumatology revised criteria *(continued)*

8. **Immunological disorder** (one of the following):
   - Anti-dsDNA: presence of antibody to native DNA in abnormal titre
   - Anti-Smith: presence of antibody to Smith nuclear antigen
   - Positive findings of antiphospholipid antibodies (anti-cardiolipin or lupus anticoagulant)
9. **Neurological disorder** (one of the following):
   - Seizures: in the absence of offending drugs or known metabolic derangements; for example, uraemia, ketoacidosis, or electrolyte imbalance
   - Psychosis: in the absence of offending drugs or known metabolic derangements; for example, uraemia, ketoacidosis, or electrolyte imbalance
10. **Malar rash** (*Fig. 2.12.3*): Fixed erythema, flat or raised, over the malar eminences, tending to spare the nasolabial folds.
11. **Discoid rash** (*Fig. 2.12.4*): Erythematous raised patches with adherent keratotic scaling and follicular plugging; atrophic scarring may occur in older lesions.

Diagnosis and investigations

Hx
- **Clinical presentation** (*see above*)
- **Family history**
- **Drug history**
- Other risk factors – sun exposure and tobacco smoking.

Ex Since any organ system can be affected in SLE, multiple organ systems need to be assessed (*Fig. 2.12.2*):

1. **Mucocutaneous**: painful / painless oral ulcers, malar rash, diffuse or patchy alopecia (*Fig. 2.12.5*) and photosensitivity (common), nasal and vaginal ulcers, and Raynaud's phenomenon (less common).
2. **Musculosketal system** (MSK): generalized arthralgia with morning stiffness is very common. Myalgia is common. Frank arthritis may involve the small joints of the hands and wrists (usually symmetrical, polyarticular and non-erosive). Deformities are very rare but include Jaccoud's arthropathy (*Fig. 2.12.6*) which occurs due to ligament laxity.
3. **Renal system**: hypertension and haematuria may be present. Oedema, weight gain and hyperlipidaemia are common physical findings related to nephrotic syndrome or volume overload with renal failure.
4. **Nervous system**: the central and peripheral nervous system should be assessed. Headache, seizures and aseptic meningitis are common.
5. **Cardiopulmonary**: pleuritis or pericarditis (*see above*).
6. **GI system**: abdominal pain, nausea, vomiting and diarrhoea can occur in up to 50% of patients with SLE.

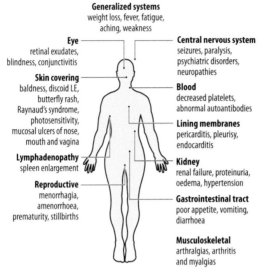

Generalized systems
weight loss, fever, fatigue, aching, weakness

Eye
retinal exudates, blindness, conjunctivitis

Skin covering
baldness, discoid LE, butterfly rash, Raynaud's syndrome, photosensitivity, mucosal ulcers of nose, mouth and vagina

Lymphadenopathy
spleen enlargement

Reproductive
menorrhagia, amenorrhoea, prematurity, stillbirths

Central nervous system
seizures, paralysis, psychiatric disorders, neuropathies

Blood
decreased platelets, abnormal autoantibodies

Lining membranes
pericarditis, pleurisy, endocarditis

Kidney
renal failure, proteinuria, oedema, hypertension

Gastrointestinal tract
poor appetite, vomiting, diarrhoea

Musculoskeletal
arthralgias, arthritis and myalgias

Fig. 2.12.2: SLE manifestations.

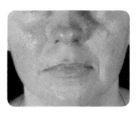

Fig. 2.12.3: Malar rash.

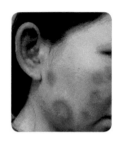

Fig. 2.12.4: Discoid rash.

Ix
- **Blood tests**:
    - FBC – anaemia, leucopenia, thrombocytopenia and rarely pancytopenia.
    - Activated prothrombin time – may be prolonged in patients with antiphospholipid antibodies.
    - ESR and CRP – elevated (non-specific).
    - Immunology – ANA antibodies, dsDNA (highly specific), Smith antigen (highly specific) positive.
    - Urea and electrolytes – elevated in renal disease.
- **Urinalysis**: haematuria, casts (red cell, granular, tubular or mixed) or proteinuria.
- **Chest X-ray**: all patients presenting with cardiopulmonary symptoms should have a chest X-ray performed for pleural effusion, infiltrates and cardiomegaly.
- **X-ray of affected joints**: periarticular osteopenia.
- **MRI**: in suspected CNS lupus.
- **ECG**: all patients presenting with cardiopulmonary symptoms should have an electrocardiogram (ECG). It may exclude other causes of chest pain.
- **Echocardiogram**: to investigate pericardial involvement.

DDx
- RA
- Antiphospholipid syndrome
- Systemic sclerosis
- Mixed connective tissue disease

Clinical facts: Complications of SLE

SLE patients are at increased risk of other serious conditions: **atherosclerosis, hypertension, dyslipidaemia, diabetes mellitus, osteoporosis, avascular necrosis, permanent neurological damage** and **lymphoma**.

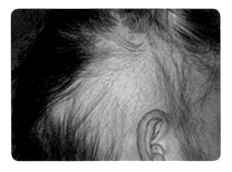

Fig. 2.12.5: Patient with alopecia.

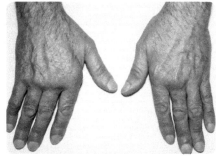

Fig. 2.12.6: Jaccoud's arthropathy.

Box 2.12.2: Antiphospholipid syndrome

Antiphospholipid syndrome may be associated with SLE but mostly exists as a primary disease. It is an important cause of recurrent arterial and venous thrombosis and miscarriages. It is associated with the presence of antiphospholipid antibodies.

Clinical features ('CLOT'):

Coagulation defects, Livedo reticularis, Obstetric (recurrent miscarriage), Thrombocytopenia.

Diagnosis (one clinical and one laboratory finding):

- Clinical – one episode of arterial and / or venous thrombosis, or morbidity in pregnancy
- Laboratory – anti-cardiolipin antibodies or lupus anticoagulant in plasma.

Management: low-dose aspirin, or warfarin if recurrent thromboses. Seek expert advice for pregnancy.

Management

Patient education

- Advice about sun exposure – patients with sun-induced rashes should use sunscreen regularly for about 6 months over the summer. Other patients with SLE should be aware that sun exposure may precipitate a flare.
- Smoking cessation.
- Pregnancy and contraception – pregnancy should be planned. Risk of problems with pregnancy is greatly reduced if disease is well controlled prior to conception. Drug therapy should be reviewed before pregnancy. Pills that contain oestrogen may exacerbate lupus disease or thrombosis and should be used with caution. In general, barrier methods or progesterone-only contraception are preferred.
- Infections should be avoided and treated promptly if appropriate.

Monitoring disease activity

- Anti-dsDNA antibody titres.
- Complement system: C3↓ C4↓, and C3d and C4d↑ suggests increased activity.

- ESR
- Others → BP, urinalysis for casts and protein, FBC, U & Es, LFTs, CRP (usually normal).

Pharmacological management

- Analgesic / NSAIDs for arthritis.
- Cardiovascular risk reduction.
- Intra-articular steroids for joint problems.
- Hydroxychloroquine for skin and joint disease.
- High-dose steroids and cyclophosphamide for patients with severe renal, cardiac or neurological involvement or associated systemic vasculitis.
- Azathioprine, methotrexate and mycophenolate are used as steroid-sparing agents.

Self-assessment

An 18 year old female presents to her GP with symptoms of fatigue, muscle pain and a facial rash. On examination she is noted to be thin with malar skin changes. No other abnormality is found. You suspect SLE.

1. What are the possible characteristic facial rashes that occur in SLE?
2. What haematological disorders may occur in SLE?
3. What autoantibodies are present in almost all patients with SLE? Which autoantibodies are most specific to SLE?
4. How can the disease activity of SLE be monitored?
5. What general advice would you give to this patient?

Answers to self-assessment questions are to be found in *Appendix A*.

Polymyositis and dermatomyositis

Polymyositis (PM) is a rare **autoimmune connective tissue disease** characterized by **inflammation** and **weakness** of **skeletal muscle**. Although PM primarily affects the muscles, it may also affect other parts of the body such as **joints**, the **oesophagus**, **lungs** and **heart**. When PM pathology extends to the **skin**, the condition is termed dermatomyositis (DM). DM may coexist with other connective tissue disorders such as SLE.

Pathophysiology

- The pathophysiology of PM and DM remains largely uncertain but both environmental and genetic factors are likely to play a part in the disease process (*Fig. 2.13.1*).

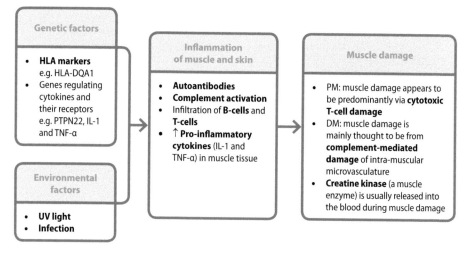

Fig. 2.13.1: Overview of the pathophysiology of PM and DM.

Epidemiology and risk factors

- PM and DM are rare – the combined incidence is approximately 2–10 cases per million each year in the general population.

Table 2.13.1: Risk factors for polymyositis and dermatomyositis	
Genetic predisposition	• There is an association between particular **HLA subtypes** and increased risk of developing PM and DM.
Age	• DM has a **bimodal age distribution** with peaks at **5–15** and **40–60 yrs**. • PM is rare in childhood and occurs mainly in adults (peak **40–60 yrs**).
Female sex	• The overall female:male ratio is **2.5:1**.
Ethnicity	• PM and DM 3 × more common in **black people** than in Caucasians.
Malignancy	• DM may occur 2° to malignancy.
Environmental factors	• **UV light**: the rash in DM often develops in sun-exposed areas and some patients report photosensitivity. • **Infections**: viruses, bacteria and protozoa have been associated with DM.

Clinical features

PM	DM (presents with PM features and dermatological features)
Commonly present with insidious, progressive and **symmetrical proximal muscle weakness** (weeks–months). The patient particularly experiences difficulties in walking up stairs or rising from a chair.	**Gottron's papules**: scaly, erythematous eruptions particularly over the extensor surfaces of the MCP, PIP and DIP joints (*Fig. 2.13.2*). Macular erythema (without scaly eruption) can occur in other extensor surfaces e.g. of the elbows and knees, known as **Gottron's sign** (*Fig. 2.13.3*).
Muscle pain (approximately 1/3).	**Heliotrope rash**: violet discoloration of the eyelids, occasionally accompanied by periorbital oedema (*Fig. 2.13.4*).
Systemic features: fever, fatigue, and weight loss (due to oesophageal dysmotility).	**Photosensitivity**
Aspiration pneumonia, **dysphagia**, **dysphonia** and **respiratory failure** (if there is involvement of the respiratory and pharyngeal muscles).	**Nail-fold erythema**
Pulmonary fibrosis (30%)	

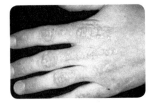
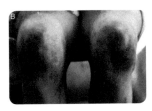
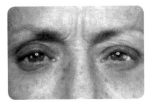

Fig. 2.13.2: Gottron's papules. Fig. 2.13.3: Gottron's sign. Fig. 2.13.4: Heliotrope rash.

Diagnosis and investigations

Hx
- See above for clinical presentation
- Risk factors e.g. family history and recent infection
- Drug history – to exclude drug-induced myopathy

Ex

Polymyositis:

- **Proximal muscle weakness** and **atrophy** occur with comparative sparing of distal muscles.
- Difficulties in arising from sitting position due to involvement of pelvic girdle muscle.
- Forced flexion of the neck is weak.
- As muscular atrophy occurs, flexor plantar response and normal sensation are maintained.
- Muscles are **tender** on palpation.

Dermatomyositis (in addition to PM clinical features):

- **Gottron's sign and papules** – present in 60–80% of DM patients.
- **Heliotrope rash** – present in ≤50%.

Ix

Blood tests:

- **Creatine kinase** (CK) – can be up to 50 x higher than normal. It is rarely normal in active disease and the level is usually a good indicator of disease activity.
- Other enzymes are ↑ – aldolase, serum glutamic-oxaloacetic transaminase (SGOT), serum glutamic-pyruvic transaminase (SGPT), and lactate dehydrogenase (LDH).
- **ESR, plasma viscosity** and **CRP** may be raised.
- Autoantibodies:
  - A positive **ANA** finding is found in approximately 60% of patients.
  - **Anti-Mi-2 antibodies** are specific for DM, but found in only 25% of patients.
  - **Anti-Jo-1 antibodies** are more common in patients with PM than in patients with DM. They are associated with interstitial lung disease, Raynaud's phenomenon and arthritis.

MRI: may show areas of inflammation in the muscle.

Electromyography (EMG): abnormal but can be normal in up to 15% of patients with DM.

Muscle biopsy: confirms diagnosis. Shows evidence of myositis.

DDx

- Drug-induced myopathy (e.g. statins)
- Mixed connective tissue disease
- Hereditary neuromuscular diseases
- SLE

OSCE tips: Malignancy in DM

DM may occur 2° to a malignancy:

- Ask about **non-specific features of malignancy** e.g. weight loss and malaise
- Perform **systems review**
- Consider performing **whole body CT, GI tract imaging** and **mammography**

Management

Non-pharmacological

- **Sun-blocking agents** should be used for DM.
- Encourage **physical activity** in order to maintain muscular strength. Involvement of a **physiotherapist** and **occupational therapist** may be beneficial.
- Evaluation of swallowing may be required. **Speech and language therapist** may help with difficulties of swallowing.
- Monitor CK levels.
- Screen thoroughly for malignancy in DM.

Pharmacological

- Start high-dose **prednisolone**: 60–80 mg/24 hours. The dose should be gradually reduced according to the clinical response of CK levels.
- **DMARDs** and **steroid-sparing drugs** can be used in early resistant cases e.g. azathioprine, methotrexate and ciclosporin.
- **Intravenous immunoglobulins** may help in some patients.
- **Hydroxychloroquine** and **tacrolimus** may help with skin disease.

Self-assessment

A 47 year old woman presents with a 5 week history of progressive weakness in her thighs and upper arms. She has difficulty getting out of a chair unaided and complains of fatigue and breathlessness. On examination, proximal muscle strength is symmetrically reduced but distal muscle strength is normal. Chest examination reveals fine bilateral basal crepitations. You suspect polymyositis.

1. What skin features help to distinguish dermatomyositis from polymyositis?
2. What blood tests would you perform on this patient and why?
3. What further definitive tests can be performed?
4. How would you measure the clinical response to treatment?

Answers to self-assessment questions are to be found in *Appendix A*.

Sjögren's syndrome

Sjögren's syndrome (SS) is an **autoimmune disorder** of unknown cause characterized by **inflammation** of the **salivary**, **lacrimal** and other **exocrine glands**. The disease is referred to as **primary** if it develops in isolation, and **secondary** if it occurs with other autoimmune diseases, usually **RA**, **SLE** or **scleroderma**.

Pathophysiology

- **Environmental** or **endogenous antigens** trigger an **immune induced inflammatory** response in **susceptible individuals**.
- The close relationship between **primary SS** and **SLE** has led to the suggestion that primary SS is likely to share similar features to the pathogenesis of SLE.
- There is particular **lymphocytic infiltration** and **fibrosis** of the **lacrimal** and **salivary glands** producing the main symptoms of **xerophthalmia** (**dry eyes**), **xerostomia** (decreased saliva production) and enlargement of the **parotid glands**.
- Other organs may also be involved but this occurs less commonly.

Epidemiology and risk factors

- The prevalence of Sjögren's syndrome in the UK is approximately 3–4%.

Table 2.14.1: Risk factors for Sjögren's syndrome	
Female	Female:male **ratio 9:1**.
SLE	Significant overlap with SS.
RA	Significant overlap with SS.
Scleroderma	Significant overlap with SS.
HLA markers	HLA class II markers -A1, -B8, or -DR3/DQ2 haplotype are linked with susceptibility to SS.
Age	Peaks at 30s–50s and after menopause.
Family history	Confers susceptibility.

Clinical features ('D factor')

- **Keratoconjunctivitis sicca** (dry eyes). ⎫
- **Xerostomia** leading to **dry mouth**. ⎬ Most common specific features
- **Parotid swelling** (*Fig. 2.14.1*). ⎭
- **Vaginal dryness** and **dyspareunia**, **dry cough** and **dysphagia** (other glands).
- **Systemic features**: polyarthritis, arthralgia, Raynaud's, lymphadenopathy, vasculitis, lung, kidney and liver involvement, peripheral neuropathy, myositis and fatigue.
- It is associated with other autoimmune diseases, e.g. SLE, and there is an increased risk of **non-Hodgkin's B-cell lymphoma**.

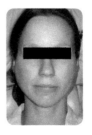

Fig. 2.14.1: Bilateral parotid swelling in SS.

Diagnosis and investigations

Hx
- **Clinical presentation**: fatigue, dry eyes and dry mouth are all common.
- **Key risk factors**: female gender, SLE, systemic sclerosis, RA, HLA type II, age (30s–50s) and post-menopause.

Ex
- **Eyes**: dilatation of the conjunctival vessels may be present. Look for corneal lesions and gently pull down the lower eyelid to assess the tear pool. Blepharitis may be present.
- **Mouth**: may look dry and a wooden tongue depressor may stick to the tongue. There may be evidence of oral candidiasis and dental caries. Submandibular glands may be enlarged but bilateral enlargement of the parotid glands is more obvious.
- **Features of other autoimmune disorders**: most commonly RA, SLE and scleroderma.

Ix
- **Schirmer's test** (*Fig. 2.14.2*): quantitatively measures tears. A filter paper is placed in the lower conjunctival sac. The test is positive if less than 5 mm of paper is wetted after 5 minutes.
- **Blood tests**:
  - Antibodies to the ribonucleoproteins 60 kD Ro (SS-A) and La (SS-B) are found in up to 90% of patients with SS.
  - Raised ESR and hypergammaglobulinaemia.
  - Positive ANA and RF.
- **Salivary gland or lip biopsy**: shows lymphocyte infiltration.
- **Lissamine green test and rose Bengal staining**: may show keratitis.
- **Salivary gland scintigraphy**: decreased salivary gland function.
- **Parotid sialography**: gross distortion of the normal pattern of parotid ductules together with significant retention of contrast material.

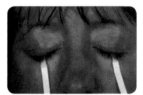

Fig. 2.14.2: Schirmer's test.

Rapid diagnosis: American–European Consensus Group classification criteria

Requires 3 of 4 objective criteria:
1. Objective ocular signs: Schirmer's test, rose Bengal testing or lissamine green and fluorescein.
2. Involvement of salivary gland by functional testing: salivary scintigraphy, parotid sialography.
3. Anti-Ro ± anti-La autoantibodies.
4. Histopathology on salivary gland biopsy.

Or 4 of 6 criteria, of which at least one of anti-Ro, anti-La, and / or histopathology must be present:
1. Objective ocular signs (i.e. Schirmer's test).
2. Involvement of salivary gland by functional testing (sialometry).
3. Autoantibodies anti-Ro or anti-La.
4. Histopathology on salivary gland biopsy.
5. Oral symptoms.
6. Ocular symptoms.

DDx	• SLE	• Salivary gland tumours
	• RA	• Sarcoidosis
	• Scleroderma	

Management

- There is no specific treatment for SS but symptoms can be contained.

Dry eyes	• **Artificial tears** are first-line therapy. • **Ophthalmic ciclosporin** drops can also be given. • **Spectacle eye shields** – a recommended adjunct to help maintain a humid environment. Also, patients should take regular breaks while reading. • **Humidifiers** – to alleviate loss of secretions by evaporation.
Dry mouth	• Patients should be encouraged to drink plenty to keep the mouth moist. • **Salivary substitutes** for improving lubrication and hydration of oral tissues are used alone as first-line therapy. • **Cholinergic drugs** to stimulate secretion of exocrine glands e.g. **pilocarpine** and **cevimeline**.
Other features	• **Vaginal lubricants** may be required and infections such as vaginal candidiasis are more likely. • **Emollients** – may benefit dry skin. • **Hydroxychloroquine** – may be useful in suppressing arthralgia and skin symptoms.

- The **Systemic Clinical Activity Index (SCAI)** has been developed to assess systemic involvement in primary SS. Factors analysed to develop the index included **fatigue**, **musculoskeletal** involvement and **Raynaud's syndrome**.

Self-assessment

A 35 year old woman presents with fatigue and a history of positive ANAs. She has had a recurrent sensation of sand in her eyes and dry mouth for over 3 months. You suspect Sjögren's syndrome.

1. What questions would you like to ask this patient?

2. What other conditions are positive for ANA?

3. What autoantibodies are specific to SS?

4. What investigation would you perform specifically for dry eyes?

5. Outline an appropriate management plan for this patient's symptoms.

Answers to self-assessment questions are to be found in *Appendix A*.

2.15 Scleroderma

Scleroderma, which is Greek for 'hard skin', is an **autoimmune** connective tissue disorder that affects the skin and other organs. There are two main types: **localized** and **systemic sclerosis (SSc)**. Localized scleroderma is more common in children and is confined to the **skin** and **subcutaneous tissue**. Systemic scleroderma may be **limited** (also known as **CREST syndrome**), which accounts for 70% of cases. The remaining 30% of cases are **diffuse**.

Pathophysiology

- The exact pathophysiology is not fully known. However, three processes are agreed to be important in disease progression:
    1. Immune system activation and development of **autoimmunity**. **ANA** is positive in 90% of patients with SSc.
    2. Up-regulation of certain cytokines (e.g. IL-1, -4, -6) contributes to **overproduction and accumulation of collagen**, which leads to hardening of the tissue.
    3. Systemic sclerosis pathology and inflammation extends to **small blood vessels**, which can result in serious comorbidities and mortality. Clinical manifestations of vasculopathy include **Raynaud's phenomenon** (see *OSCE tips*), digital ulcers, renal crisis (accompanied by hypertension), pulmonary hypertension, and abnormalities in nail fold capillaries.

Epidemiology and risk factors

- The UK prevalence is 1:10 000.
- Although systemic sclerosis is rare, it has a high mortality rate.

Table 2.15.1: Risk factors for scleroderma	
Positive ANA	• 90% of patients with SSc are positive for **serum ANA**.
Family history	• First-degree family history of SSc increases the risk by 60%.
Gender	• Female:male ratio is **4:1**.
Age	• Localized scleroderma is more common in children and young adults. SSc is more common in older adults.
Environmental factors	• Triggering factors may include **cytomegalovirus** and **chemicals**. Exposure to **silica dust** is associated with **limited SSc**.

Clinical features

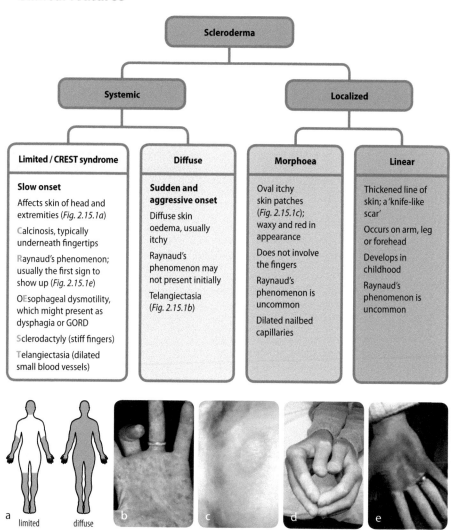

Fig. 2.15.1: **(a)** Skin involvement distribution in SSc; **(b)** Telangiectasia (red spots); **(c)** Oval morphoea skin patch; **(d)** Prayer sign (unable to contact palmar surfaces together); **(e)** Raynaud's phenomenon (white / ischaemic colour stage).

- Raynaud's phenomenon is the first symptom in nearly all patients with SSc (especially limited SSc); the next symptoms usually appear within two years.
- **Skin thickness** is reliable diagnostic clinical sign; usually starts as **swelling and puffiness** of the skin (typically in the hands).
- SSc can affect internal organs:
  - Lung → **pulmonary hypertension**, due to blood vessel damage, is a leading cause of mortality in patients with **limited SSc**. Overproduction of collagen can lead to **interstitial lung disease (diffuse SSc)**.

- Heart → **right heart failure** and **pericardial effusions**.
- Kidney → **renal impairment**.

OSCE tips: Raynaud's phenomenon
WHITE → BLUE → RED!

- **Transient vasospasm** of the peripheral blood vessels (typically in the digits) leading to hypoxia. In extreme conditions it can cause **ischaemic gangrene** and **digital ulcers**.
- It is a common condition which affects 1–3% of population.
- **Stress** and **cold** are classic triggers of the phenomenon.
- Two types:
  - **Primary** (Raynaud's disease) which accounts for 90% of cases.
  - **Secondary** (10%) – usually due to connective tissue disorders such as SSc.
- Clinically diagnosed → **digits change colour** from **white** to **blue** to **red**.

Diagnosis and investigations

Hx
- Nature of **onset** and **duration** of signs and symptoms are key.
- CREST syndrome → may present as gastro-oesophageal reflux disease (GORD, heartburn), dysphagia (liquids and solids), and weight loss.
- Risk factors including **family history** and **environmental factors**.

Ex
- Raynaud's phenomenon → initial sign for SSc.
- Hand swelling and stiffness due to thickened or hardened skin (worse in morning) → reduced range of movement (prayer sign; *Fig. 2.15.1d*).
- Note the extent of skin involvement.
- Subcutaneous calcinosis and telangiectasia.
- Foot swelling → prompt CVS examination (heart failure) and kidney function tests (renal impairment).
- Respiratory system examination → interstitial lung disease signs.

Ix **Blood tests**:
- Haematology – usually normal.
  - ESR and WCC may be raised.
  - Anaemia of chronic disease.
- Immunology:
  - **ANA** – found in up to 90% of patients but lacks specificity.
  - **Anti-topoisomerase-1 (Scl 70)** antibody – associated with lung fibrosis and renal disease in both subsets of systemic sclerosis.
  - **Anti-centromere antibody (ACA)** – only in patients with CREST syndrome.
  - **Anti-RNA polymerase I and III antibody** – associated with diffuse scleroderma, especially with kidney involvement.
- Biochemistry:
  - Blood urea and creatinine – elevated in renal impairment.

Respiratory (lung involvement is major cause of mortality in SSc):
- Complete pulmonary function test – interstitial lung disease and pulmonary hypertension.
- Chest X-ray – interstitial lung disease, enlarged pulmonary arteries or enlarged right ventricle.
- High resolution CT – interstitial lung disease.

Cardiovascular system: echocardiogram shows raised pulmonary artery pressure and right ventricle dysfunction.

Gastrointestinal: barium swallow test (oesophageal dysmotility).

DDx
- Primary Raynaud's
- Other secondary causes of Raynaud's
- Other connective tissue disorders or mixed connective tissue disorders
- Scleromyxoedema
- Paraneoplastic syndromes

Management

Specific management is formulated dependent on the organ involved:

Skin	Skin hygiene and use of emollients for dry skin.
	Low-dose **prednisolone** or **methotrexate** (if synovitis is associated).
Vascular	Avoiding triggering factors for Raynaud's phenomenon.
	For Raynaud's use one of the following vasodilators: • **Phosphodiesterase type 5 (PDE5) inhibitors** • **Endothelin-1 receptor antagonists (ERA)** • **Prostacyclin agonists** • **Calcium channel blockers**
Gastrointestinal	Avoid eating 2–3 hours before bedtime and avoid caffeine.
	PPI inhibitors or **H2-receptor agonists** for exacerbated conditions.
	Antibiotics for signs of GI infection (diarrhoea, unintentional weight loss and malabsorption).
Renal disease	An angiotension-converting enzyme (**ACE**) **inhibitor** for patients at risk of renal crisis.
Cardiac	Oral prednisolone + close monitoring of blood pressure (cardiac tamponade) for patients with pericardial effusion.
	Patients with cardiac tamponade require urgent medical care.
Pulmonary hypertension	ERA, PDE5 inhibitor or prostacyclin agonists.
Respiratory	**Cyclophosphamide** for patients with interstitial lung disease. The main disadvantage is that it increases patient's risk of infection.

Self-assessment

A 39 year old woman complains of distal finger pain and tightening. She also has a history of Raynaud's for the past 4 years.

1. What clinical feature is illustrated in the patient's finger (*Fig. 2.15.2*)?
2. What is the most likely diagnosis?
3. What other signs would you look for during examination?
4. Which serum autoantibodies is she mostly likely to be positive for?

The patient revisits you after 6 months complaining of difficulty breathing.

5. What is the most likely underlying cause of her symptoms and what further investigations will you perform?

Answers to self-assessment questions are to be found in *Appendix A*.

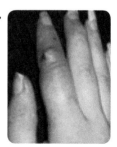

Fig. 2.15.2: Skin changes affecting the hand.

Fibromyalgia

Fibromyalgia is a syndrome of **chronic pain** and the presence of **hyperalgesic points** at specific anatomical sites, as well as a range of other **physical** and **psychological symptoms** with **no identifiable organic cause**.

Pathophysiology

The cause of fibromyalgia is poorly understood but **abnormal central** and **peripheral pain processing** is thought to be responsible for **reduced pain threshold**, **hyperalgesia** (amplification of pain) and **allodynia** (pain produced by a non-noxious stimulus).

Epidemiology and risk factors

- The prevalence of fibromyalgia in the general population is approximately 2–4%, but it is a condition that is underdiagnosed.
- The incidence of fibromyalgia in primary care in the UK is approximately 14 700 new cases per year.
- There are recognized risk factors for fibromyalgia but they only contribute approximately 5–10% to disease development (*Table 2.16.1*).

Table 2.16.1: Risk factors for fibromyalgia	
Gender	• **10** × more common in **women** than men.
Age	• More common in individuals **aged 20–50**.
Physical trauma	• For example **whiplash type injuries** to the **neck** and **trunk**.
Psychological trauma	• **Stress, anxiety** and **depression**.
Viral infections	• May occur as a **post-viral syndrome**.

Clinical features

'Fibro':

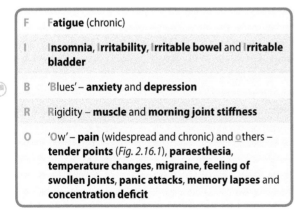

F	**Fatigue** (chronic)
I	**Insomnia, Irritability, Irritable bowel** and **Irritable bladder**
B	'Blues' – **anxiety** and **depression**
R	Rigidity – **muscle** and **morning joint stiffness**
O	'Ow' – **pain** (widespread and chronic) and others – **tender points** (*Fig. 2.16.1*), **paraesthesia, temperature changes, migraine, feeling of swollen joints, panic attacks, memory lapses** and **concentration deficit**

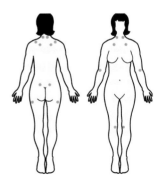

Fig. 2.16.1: Distribution of hyperalgesic tender points.

Diagnosis and investigations

Hx
- See above for symptoms and risk factors.
- A full **social**, **personal**, **family** and **psychological history** should be taken to reveal any past **physical trauma** or **psychological disturbance**.

Ex
- **Widespread pain**, above and below the waist as well as the axial skeletal system, for at least **3 months**.
- The presence of **11/18 tender points** shown in *Fig. 2.16.1*.
- **Digital palpation** using the thumb to assess tender points. The pressure applied should be just enough to blanch the examiner's thumbnail. In the absence of fibromyalgia, the palpation would not be enough to cause pain.

Ix
- **Blood tests** → normal
  - Haematology
  - Biochemistry
  - Immunology
- **Imaging** → normal

Yellow flags: Psychosocial risk factors for developing persisting chronic pain and long-term disability

- Belief that pain and activity are harmful
- Demonstration of sickness behaviour e.g. prolonged rest
- Withdrawal from society
- Emotional problems – low mood, anxiety and stress
- Problems or dissatisfaction at work
- Problems with claims for compensation or time off work
- Overprotective family or lack of social support
- Inappropriate expectations of treatment

DDx
- Chronic fatigue syndrome (myalgic encephalomyelitis)
- Hypothyroidism
- Polymyalgia rheumatica
- Polymyositis

Rapid diagnosis: A typical fibromyalgia patient

- A **30–50 year old female** patient with a **long-standing history** of **diffuse pain**.
- She may have a history of **physical** or **psychological trauma**.
- The symptoms are **constant** but are exacerbated by certain stressors.
- She may not have received treatment from previous doctors based on **normal investigation findings**.
- This may have exacerbated her symptoms by causing further **anxiety** and possibly even **depression**.
- On examination **hyperalgesic points** that are **tender to palpate** may be demonstrated.

Management (based on EULAR recommendations, 2008)

General points	
• Pain and function should be assessed in a psychosocial context.	
• Access to a **multidisciplinary team** with treatments taking into account the **patient's needs** including **pain intensity**, **function**, **depression**, **fatigue** and **sleep disturbance**.	
Non-pharmacological	
Heated pool treatment	Can improve pain and function with or without exercise.
Exercise programmes	Individually tailored exercise programmes which include **aerobic training** and **muscle strengthening**.
Cognitive behavioural therapy (CBT)	A form of **psychotherapy** that is based on scientific principles that help people change the way they think, feel and behave.
Others	**Relaxation**, **rehabilitation**, **physiotherapy** and **psychological support**.
Pharmacological	
Tramadol	A **moderate opioid** which is recommended for pain management.
Mild pain relief	**Paracetamol** and weak opioids such as **codeine** can also be considered.
Antidepressants	Reduce pain and improve function e.g. **fluoxetine** and **amitriptyline**.
Pramipexole and pregabalin	Relatively new treatments which reduce pain.

Self-assessment

A 40 year old woman complains of muscle pain all over the body and lack of sleep. On examination, tender symmetrical spots are identified on multiple sites.

1. What is the most likely diagnosis?
2. What would you expect to see if routine blood tests are performed?
3. Name two non-pharmacological approaches which can be offered.
4. Name suitable mild and moderate forms of pain relief for this patient.

Answers to self-assessment questions are to be found in *Appendix A*.

Osteoporosis is a **progressive**, **systemic skeletal disorder** characterized by **low bone mass** and **micro-architectural deterioration** of **bone tissue**, with a resultant increase in **bone fragility** and susceptibility to **fracture**. Osteoporosis exists when **bone mineral density (BMD)** values are reduced by more than **2.5 standard deviations** below that observed in **young healthy adults**.

Pathophysiology

- The underlying cause of osteoporosis is excessive **bone resorption** by **osteoclast cells** at a rate that exceeds **bone formation** by **osteoblast cells**.
- This results in **decreased bone mass** and **incomplete bone remodelling**.
- **Oestrogen deficiency** as a result of **menopause** is the commonest cause of osteoporosis.
- **Oestrogen deficiency** → ↑ production of **RANK ligand (RANK-L)** by **osteoblasts** → ↑ **osteoclast formation, function** and **survival** → ↑ **osteoclastic activity** → ↑ **bone resorption** → ↓ **BMD**.
- Individuals with **inherited low peak bone mass, impaired absorption of calcium** and other coexisting **metabolic bone diseases** such as **hyperparathyroidism** →↑ risk of osteoporosis.
- Long-term use of **glucocorticoid therapy** ↓ **osteoblastic activity** → ↑ risk of osteoporosis.
- Based on the **pattern of bone loss** and **fracture**, osteoporosis can be classified (*Fig. 2.17.1*) as:

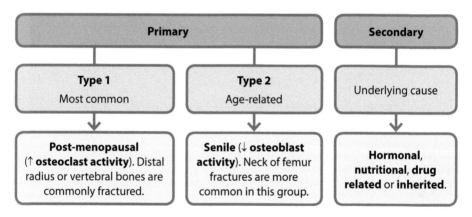

Fig. 2.17.1: Classification of osteoporosis.

Epidemiology and risk factors

- It is estimated that over **200 million people** have **osteoporosis worldwide**.
- There are approximately **2.8 million people** with osteoporosis in the **UK**.
- Risk factors include **female sex, family history** and 'SHATTERED':

S	**Steroid use**, **Smoking**
H	**Hypo / Hyperthyroidism**, **Hyperparathyroidism**, **Hypercalcinuria**
A	**Age** (>50), **Alcohol**
T	**Thin** (BMI <22)
T	**Testosterone deficiency**
E	**Early menopause**
R	**Renal, liver failure**
E	**Erosive bone disease**, e.g. RA or myeloma
D	**Deficiency of calcium and / or vitamin D**, **Diabetes**

Clinical features

- Usually **asymptomatic**.
- Clinical signs arise with fractures which commonly occur in the **spine** (*Fig. 2.17.2*), **hip** (*Fig. 2.17.3*) and **wrist** (*Fig. 2.17.4*):
  - **Back pain**, **reduced height**, **kyphosis** and **respiratory difficulty** (vertebral fracture).
  - **Painful**, **shortened** and **externally rotated hip** (hip fracture).
  - **Pain** and **deformity** (wrist / other fractures).

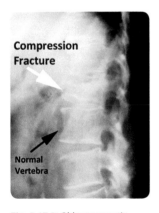

Fig. 2.17.2: Old osteoporotic compression fracture.

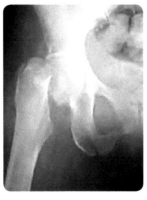

Fig. 2.17.3: Intra-capsular neck of femur fracture.

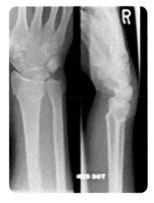

Fig. 2.17.4: Colles' wrist fracture.

Diagnosis and investigations

Hx	- Usually **asymptomatic** unless a fracture is present.
	- Ask about **risk factors**, e.g. **steroid use**, **family history** and **menopause**.

Ex
- **Height loss** and **kyphosis** (vertebral fracture).
- **Painful**, **shortened** and **externally rotated hip** (hip fracture).
- **Pain** and **deformity** (other fractures).

Ix

Blood tests:
- ↑ **Parathyroid hormone (PTH) levels** → **hyperparathyroidism**
- **Thyroid function tests (TFT)** → ↓ **T3, T4 (hypothyroidism)** ↑ **T3, T4 (hyperthyroidism)**
- ↑ **Serum FSH**, ↓ **sex hormones**, ↓ **androgens** → **sex hormone deficiency / menopause**.
- ↓ **Vitamin D** → **vitamin D deficiency**
- ↑ **ESR** → **inflammatory disease** e.g. **RA** or **myeloma**
- **Bone biomarkers**, e.g. **calcium** and **alkaline phosphate** are usually normal

X-ray: to **confirm fracture** (if suspected); cannot determine if patient has osteoporosis but can predict if bones are **osteopenic**.

Dual-energy X-ray absorptiometry (DEXA) scan: works out the **BMD** of the patient in the **spine** and **hip**; two scores are calculated:
- **T-score** → diagnostic of osteoporosis; gives the number of **standard deviations** the **BMD** is from a **young healthy adult** (*Table 2.17.1*)
- **Z-score** → compares an individual's results to others of the **same age** and **gender**; a **Z-score of <−1.5** raises concern of factors other than ageing contributing to osteoporosis.

DDx
- Osteomalacia
- Paget's disease
- Hyperparathyroidism
- Multiple myeloma

Table 2.17.1: WHO osteoporosis criteria	
T-score	**Interpretation**
>0	BMD better than reference population
0 to −1	No evidence of osteoporosis
−1 to −2.5	Osteopenia
−2.5 or below	Osteoporosis
−2.5 or below plus fracture	Established osteoporosis

Clinical facts: Osteoporosis
- Osteoporotic fractures cause significant **morbidity** and ↑ the likelihood of **mortality**.
- **Hip fractures** have the **highest morbidity** and **mortality**, with **20–30%** of patients dying within the **first year** of fracture.
- The **Fracture Risk Assessment Tool (FRAX)** can be used to predict fractures based on **clinical risk factors**, with or without the use of **femoral neck bone mineral density**.

Management

Non-pharmacological management

Smoking cessation and **reduction** in **alcohol** consumption, weight-bearing muscle **exercises**, **dietary** (adequate source of **calcium** and **vitamin D**), **physiotherapy**, assessment of home **safety** and reducing the risk of falls (especially in the elderly).

Pharmacological management

See *Table 2.17.2*.

Table 2.17.2: Pharmacological management of osteoporosis based on National Institute for Health and Care Excellence (NICE) recommendations (2012)

Bisphosphonates	First-line. **Inhibit bone resorption** by **inhibiting osteoclasts**. Examples include **alendronate** (**first-line**), **risedronate** and **zoledronate**. Can be taken orally once a week (alendronate) or as once-yearly IV injections (zoledronate). **GI side-effects** are common with oral medication and patients are asked to sit or stand for at least 30 minutes to reduce side-effects of **oesophagitis**.
Denosumab	**Monoclonal antibodies** directed against **RANK-L**. Used as an alternative treatment to bisphosphonates. Given as **6-monthly injections**.
Strontium ranelate	Mechanism of action unknown but thought to **stimulate osteoblasts** and **inhibit osteoclasts (dual action)**. Taken **once daily in water** (preferably at **bedtime**). Used as an alternative to bisphosphonates. Side-effects: **nausea, diarrhoea, headache, dizziness**. Limited use because of risk of **DVT** and **thromboembolism**.
Teriparatide	A **parathyroid hormone analogue**. **Intermittent** exposure to **parathyroid hormone** activates **osteoblasts** more than **osteoclasts** and thus stimulates **new bone formation**. Taken as a **once-daily injection** into the **thigh or abdomen**. Very **expensive**. Used in very **severe cases**.
Other	**Raloxifene, calcitonin, hormone replacement therapy (HRT)** – these are less commonly used.

Self-assessment

A 32 year old man being treated for sarcoidosis develops back pain 6 months after steroid treatment was commenced. The radiologist reports a vertebral crush fracture and suggests that the 'bones look osteopenic in nature'. A diagnosis of osteoporosis is later confirmed.

1. What is the mechanism by which osteoporosis has been caused?
2. How could this have been prevented?
3. What first-line treatment would you prescribe? Name the most common side-effects.

A 43 year old woman has been complaining of amenorrhoea and hot flushes. The patient is later diagnosed with premature ovarian failure. A routine DEXA scan is performed and T-scores of −2.2 and −1.3 are reported in the vertebrae and hip, respectively.

4. What do the T-scores reveal in this patient?

5. What blood tests would you like to perform and why?

6. What lifestyle advice would you recommend to this lady?

Answers to self-assessment questions are to be found in *Appendix A*.

2.18 Paget's disease

Paget's disease is a common bone disease characterized by focal increases in bone remodelling, resulting in the **abnormal production of bone** which is **mechanically weak**. The most commonly affected bones include the **pelvis**, **spine**, **skull**, **femur** and **tibia**.

Pathophysiology

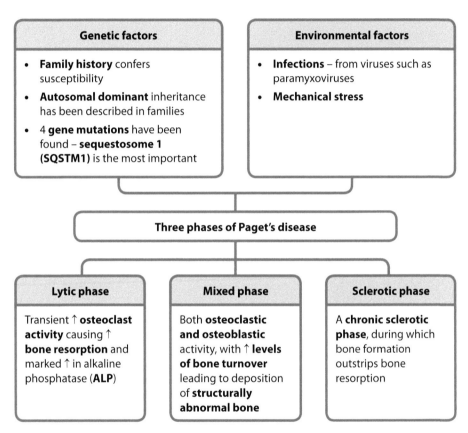

Genetic factors

- **Family history** confers susceptibility
- **Autosomal dominant** inheritance has been described in families
- 4 **gene mutations** have been found – **sequestosome 1 (SQSTM1)** is the most important

Environmental factors

- **Infections** – from viruses such as paramyxoviruses
- **Mechanical stress**

Three phases of Paget's disease

Lytic phase

Transient ↑ **osteoclast activity** causing ↑ **bone resorption** and marked ↑ in alkaline phosphatase (**ALP**)

Mixed phase

Both **osteoclastic and osteoblastic** activity, with ↑ **levels of bone turnover** leading to deposition of **structurally abnormal bone**

Sclerotic phase

A **chronic sclerotic phase**, during which bone formation outstrips bone resorption

Fig. 2.18.1: Outline of the pathophysiology of Paget's disease.

Epidemiology and risk factors

- The UK has the highest prevalence of Paget's disease in the world – approximately 2% in Caucasians over the age of 55.
- The condition is very rare in Asians.

Table 2.18.1: Risk factors for Paget's disease	
Age	• The mean age of onset is approximately **55 years**.
Gender	• The male:female ratio is **2:1**.
Ethnicity	• Common in the UK but very rare in Asian countries.
Family history	• The relative risk can be **up to 7-fold** in **first-degree relatives** of patients with Paget's disease.

Clinical features

- Paget's disease is usually **asymptomatic** (**70–90%**) and therefore diagnosed on incidental abnormal X-ray or biochemical findings (↑ **ALP**).
- Complications depend on the site affected as well as the activity of the disease (*Table 2.18.2*).

Table 2.18.2: Typical complications of Paget's disease	
Bone pain	Most common
Bone deformity & enlargement	Typically the pelvis, lumbar spine, skull, femur and tibia (*Fig. 2.18.2*)
↑ Temperature over affected bone	Due to hypervascularity
Pathological fractures	Due to mechanically weak bone
2° OA	Due to Paget's disease surrounding the joint
Hearing loss and tinnitus	If Paget's disease affects the skull bones and compresses the vestibulocochlear nerve

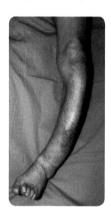

Fig. 2.18.2: Clinical bowing of the tibia in Paget's disease.

- **Less common complications**: spinal stenosis, nerve compression syndromes and cauda equina syndrome.
- **Rare complications**: hypercalcaemia, high output cardiac failure, paraplegia and osteosarcoma.

Diagnosis and investigations

Hx
- Usually **asymptomatic** but **bone pain, pathological fractures, deformities, ↑ local temperature** and **hearing loss** are all common.
- **Family history**.

Ex
- Look for head signs – ↑ **skull size**, **frontal bossing**, **deep-set eyes**, **large maxilla** with **prominent arches**.
- Look for other deformities such as **bowing** of **long bones** and **kyphosis**.
- Feel for **temperature** over affected bone.
- **Weber's** and **Rinne's test** – to elicit possible **sensorineural** hearing loss.
- Signs of other complications such as **OA** and **spinal cord compression**.

Ix
- **Blood tests**: ↑ **ALP**, **bone-specific ALP** (if known liver disease), phosphate and calcium are normal.
- **X-ray**: (*Figs 2.18.3* and *2.18.4*): **localized enlargement**, **patchy cortical thickening** with **sclerosis**, **osteolysis** and deformity, **advancing lytic lesion** in the long bones.
- **MRI**: for suspected spinal stenosis and cord compression.

DDx
- Osteomalacia
- Osteoporosis
- Fibrous dysplasia
- Myeloma

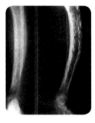

Fig. 2.18.3: X-ray showing the 'sabre tibia' in Paget's disease.

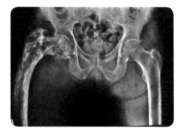

Fig. 2.18.4: X-ray of Paget's disease of the femur.

Management

Conservative management
- Observation, regular follow-up, patient education and preventive measures.
- Orthotic **devices**, **sticks** and **walkers** may be useful for Paget's disease of the legs.
- Adequate intake of **calcium** and **vitamin D**.

Pharmacological management
- Main indication is bone pain.
- **Bisphosphonates** to reduce bone turnover e.g. oral risedronate or IV zoledronate.
- **NSAIDs** and **paracetamol** for pain relief.

Surgical management
- Bone deformity, osteoarthritis, pathological fractures and nerve compression may necessitate surgery.
- Surgical procedures include **fracture fixation** (pathological fracture), **joint replacement** (secondary OA), and **osteotomy** (deformity).

Self-assessment

A 50 year old man complains of constantly aching legs. Blood tests reveal an elevated level of serum ALP. Subsequent X-ray of the tibia shows a degree of tibial bowing. You suspect Paget's disease.

1. List some risk factors for Paget's disease.
2. What other bones are commonly affected in Paget's disease?
3. Apart from bone pain, name five other complications that can arise from Paget's disease.
4. How should this patient be managed pharmacologically?
5. How would you monitor the response to treatment?

Answers to self-assessment questions are to be found in *Appendix A*.

Chapter 3

Paediatric rheumatology conditions

3.1   Vitamin D deficiency   86
3.2   Juvenile idiopathic arthritis   91

3.1 Vitamin D deficiency

Vitamin D deficiency (also known as **hypovitaminosis D**) remains one of the most common vitamin deficiencies. It causes **inadequate mineralization of bone** and clinically manifests as **rickets** in children and **osteomalacia** in adults.

Pathophysiology

- Normal bone mineralization depends on adequate **calcium** and **phosphate** and this is maintained by vitamin D.
- **Vitamin D deficiency** is most commonly caused by failure of the kidneys to **hydroxylate 25-hydroxyvitamin D (25-OHD)** to **1,25-dihydroxyvitamin D** (due to **chronic kidney disease**), and from **inadequate ultraviolet B sunlight exposure** for the formation of vitamin D_3 in skin.
- This results in ↓ **mineralization of bone** via an ↑ **parathyroid hormone (PTH)** in response to ↓ **circulating levels of phosphate and calcium** (*Fig. 3.1.1*).
- Other causes of vitamin D deficiency are also shown in *Box 3.1.1*.

> **Box 3.1.1:** Causes of vitamin D deficiency
>
> - **Lack of sunlight** – especially those who routinely cover their face and hands (e.g. Muslim women) and those who are housebound (e.g. elderly individuals)
> - **Renal disease** – due to impairment of C-1 hydroxylation of 25-OHD
> - **GI malabsorption – coeliac disease, short bowel syndrome** and **cystic fibrosis**
> - **Liver disease** – due to impaired C-25 hydroxylation of vitamin D
> - **Drugs** – use of **anticonvulsants, rifampicin, cholestyramine, highly active antiretroviral treatment (HAART)**, or **glucocorticoids**
> - **Genetic causes – hypophosphotaemic rickets, type 1** (impaired C-1 hydroxylation) and **type 2 vitamin D resistance rickets** (target organ resistance).

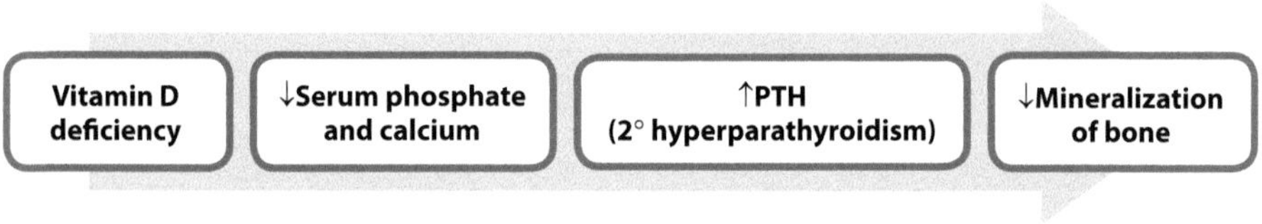

Vitamin D deficiency	↓Serum phosphate and calcium	↑PTH (2° hyperparathyroidism)	↓Mineralization of bone

Fig. 3.1.1: Overview of the pathophysiology of rickets / osteomalacia.

Epidemiology and risk factors

- Approximately 1 billion people worldwide have vitamin D deficiency.
- Over 50% of adults in the UK have insufficient levels of vitamin D.

Table 3.1.1: Risk factors for vitamin D deficiency	
Dark skin	• **Afro-Caribbean, Middle Eastern** and **south Asians.**
Age	• **Children** and those **over 65 years.**
Breastfeeding	• Infants who are exclusively breastfed.
Obesity	• When BMI is >30, fat sequesters vitamin D.
Routine covering of face and hands	• Common among **Muslim women** who wear veils.
Housebound	• Limited exposure to sunlight – particularly the **elderly.**
Sunscreen	• **Skin-concealing garments** or **strict sunscreen** use.
Pregnancy	• Multiple, short interval pregnancies.

Clinical features

Rickets	Osteomalacia
Infants: **growth retardation**, **hypotonia** and **apathy.**	**Bone pain** and **tenderness.**
Once walking: **knock-kneed** (genu valgum; *Fig. 3.1.2*); **bow-legged** (genu varum; *Fig. 3.1.3*); **deformities of the metaphyseal–epiphyseal junction.**	**Pathological fractures** (particularly femoral neck).
Hypocalcaemia (severe vitamin D deficiency) – paraesthesia, tetany, cramps, seizures.	**Proximal myopathy** causing proximal weakness and possibly a waddling gait.

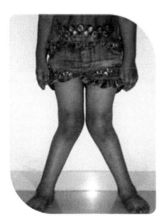

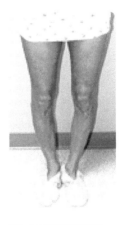

Fig. 3.1.2: Genu valgum.　　　　Fig. 3.1.3: Genu varum.

Diagnosis and investigation

Hx
- Explore **risk factors**.
- *Rickets* → failure to thrive, delayed achievement of motor milestones, fatigue and malaise, bowing of the legs, delayed tooth eruption and dental caries, chest deformity, and head sweating are all common.
- *Osteomalacia* → localized or generalized bone tenderness and muscle weakness.

Ex
- *Rickets* → bowing of the legs, widening of the bones, chest deformity and more (*Fig. 3.1.4*).
- *Osteomalacia* → bone tenderness (particularly in the back, pelvis and long bones of the leg), proximal muscle weakness and waddling gait, pathological fractures, and signs of hypocalcaemia.

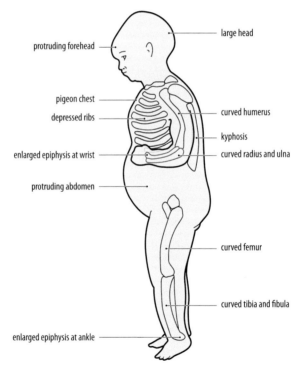

Fig. 3.1.4: Bone deformities in children with rickets.

Ix **Blood tests:**

- ↓ **25 hydroxyvitamin D** (<25 nmol/L)
- → ↓ **Ca²⁺**
- ↑ **PTH**
- ↓ **fasting phosphate**
- →↑ **ALP**

X-rays (of weight-bearing bones):

- *Osteomalacia:*

  - **Pseudofractures or Looser zones** are pathognomonic of osteomalacia. They are low-density bands extending from the cortex inwards in the shafts of long bones (*Fig. 3.1.5*)
  - **Coarse trabeculae**
  - **Osteopenia**

- *Rickets:*

  - **Metaphyseal cupping** and **flaring**
  - **Epiphyseal irregularities**
  - **Widening of the epiphyseal plates**

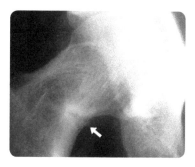

Fig. 3.1.5: Looser zone (arrow) seen in the femoral neck of a patient with osteomalacia.

DDx

- Primary hyperparathyroidism
- Osteoporosis
- Multiple myeloma
- Paget's disease

Management

General measures:

- Treat the **underlying cause**.
- **Adequate sun exposure** – advise patients to sit in the sun.
- **Adequate dietary intake of vitamin D** – foods such as oily fish / cod liver oil, egg yolk and milk are rich in vitamin D. Some foods are supplemented with vitamin D, such as breakfast cereals.
- **Daily vitamin D and calcium tablets, e.g. Adcal D₃.**

Box 3.1.2: Implications of vitamin D deficiency / insufficiency

Vitamin D deficiency is also associated with adverse health risks including:

- ↑ risk of **type 2 diabetes mellitus**
- ↑ risk of **several cancers,** e.g. prostate cancer
- ↑ risk of **cardiovascular disease**

Supplementation:

In patients with developed vitamin deficiency (25-OHD <25 nmol/L), high-dose supplementation is needed to achieve adequate vitamin D replacement (*Table 3.1.2*).

Table 3.1.2: High-dose vitamin D supplementation in children and adults	
Children	**Adults**
<6 months old – **3000 IU oral calciferol daily** for **8–12 weeks** with calcium supplementation, followed by **200–400 IU calciferol** daily maintenance.	**10 000 IU calciferol daily** or **60 000 IU calciferol weekly** for **8–12 weeks** followed by **1000–2000 IU calciferol daily maintenance** (10 000 IU weekly).
>6 months old – **6000 IU oral calciferol** daily for **8–12 weeks** followed by **400–800 IU calciferol daily.**	Patients with severe malabsorption are treated with **intramuscular calciferol 300 000 IU monthly for 3 months** and then yearly maintenance doses.

Self-assessment

A 2 year old girl has failure to thrive and an unusual gait. She has bowed legs and thick wrists. Her weight and height are below that expected for her age. Her diet consists predominantly of breastfeeding 5 times daily. Laboratory studies reveal the 25-hydroxyvitamin D level is decreased.

1. What condition is this girl suffering from?
2. What is the cause of her condition?
3. What further blood tests would you request?
4. What abnormalities do you expect to see on X-ray of her wrists and knees?
5. Her parents are extremely worried. How would you reassure them?

Answers to self-assessment questions are to be found in *Appendix A*.

Juvenile idiopathic arthritis

By definition, juvenile idiopathic arthritis (JIA) is defined as any chronic (**≥6 weeks**) **arthritis** affecting individuals **under the age of 16 years** with other known conditions excluded.

Pathophysiology

- The pathophysiology of JIA is poorly understood.
- Monozygotic twin concordance (25–40%) indicates the importance of genetic factors.
- Different HLA polymorphisms have been associated with different subtypes of JIA; these include **HLA-B27 (enthesitis-related JIA)** and **HLA-DR5 (oligoarticular)**.
- **Systemic JIA** is characterized by **chronic inflammation** of the **synovium** with infiltration of inflammatory cells. These then release various pro-inflammatory cytokines (e.g. TNF-alpha) which favours a TH-1 type response.
- This results in **increased synovial fluid production** and a **thickened synovial lining**.
- According to the International League of Associations for Rheumatology (ILAR), JIA can be classified into seven subtypes (*Table 3.2.1*).

Table 3.2.1: ILAR classification of JIA

Sub-group	Prevalence %
1) Oligoarticular JIA	50
2) Polyarticular JIA – RF negative	25
3) Polyarticular JIA – RF positive	5
4) Systemic-onset JIA	5–10
5) Juvenile psoriatic arthritis	2–15
6) Enthesitis-related arthritis	2–10
7) Undifferentiated arthritis	1–10

Epidemiology and risk factors

- Overall prevalence of JIA is estimated to be 1–2 per 1000 children in the UK.
- The incidence of JIA is 1 per 10 000 in the UK.
- JIA is more common in females (2:1).

Table 3.2.2: Risk factors for JIA

Gender	• More common in girls (**2:1**).
Age	• More common in children **aged 2–3**.
Genetic	• **HLA-B27** (enthesitis-related JIA) and **HLA-DR5** (oligoarticular).
Family history	• Family history of **psoriasis** (first-degree relative), **ankylosing spondylitis** and **inflammatory bowel disease.**

Clinical presentation

Subtype	Presentation
Oligoarthritis	• *Definition*: arthritis affecting 1–4 joints in the first six months • *Persisting oligoarthritis*: **>4 joints** affected within **6 months** • *Extending oligoarthritis*: **<4 joints** affected within **6 months** • More common in young girls (under the age of 6) • Classically presents with one or two swollen joints causing stiffness and reduced range of movement • **ANA** is positive in 70% • There is no systemic upset and RF is negative • Most commonly affects the **knee** and **ankle** • Prognosis is good for persisting but poor for extending
Polyarticular RF negative	• *Definition*: **≥5 joints** affected within **6 months** with a **negative rheumatoid factor** • 2 peaks of age: **toddler to preschool age** and **pre-adolescent** • More common in females (ratio 3:1) • May be **asymmetrical** – high risk of uveitis • May be **symmetrical** with both large and small joint swelling • Presents with minimal swelling but increased stiffness • Often destructive in nature • High remission rate (25%)
Polyarticular RF positive	• *Definition*: **≥5 joints** affected in the **first 6 months** with a **positive RF** seen on two separate occasions • More common in older girls (>8 years) • Associated with **HLA-DR4** • **Symmetrical involvement** of **small joints**, particularly the **hands** and **wrists** with swelling and stiffness • **Erosions**, **joint destruction, rheumatoid nodules** and **systemic features**, e.g. fever and lymphadenopathy • Low remission rate (6%)
Systemic arthritis (Still's disease)	• *Definition*: arthritis with **intermittent fever ≥2 weeks**. There must be one or more of the following: • **Maculopapular rash** (salmon colour which quickly fades) • **Lymphadenopathy** • **Hepatomegaly** and / or **splenomegaly** • **Serositis** (pericarditis, pleuritis, peritonitis) • Males and females (1:1), usually before **5 years of age** • Arthritis only seen at disease onset in 1/3 of children but commonly develops within a few months, usually symmetrical in nature and affecting several joints • Recurrence is common

Subtype	Presentation
Juvenile psoriatic arthritis	• *Definition*: **arthritis and psoriasis or arthritis** plus at least two of: • **Dactylitis** • **Nail pitting** or **onycholysis** • **Psoriasis** in a first-degree relative • Female: male ratio (2:1) • Mean age of onset 6 years • **Asymmetrical arthritis** affecting **small and large joints** • Psoriasis usually occurs before arthritis (>50%) • Prognosis moderate
Enthesitis-related JIA	• *Definition*: **arthritis** or **enthesitis** plus two of: • **Sacroiliac** or **lumbosacral pain** • **HLA-B27-positive** • **Family history of HLA-B27-related disease** • **Acute anterior uveitis** • Onset in a **male >6 years of age** • Male: female ratio (9:1) • Usually presents in those over 10 years • Prognosis is moderate, with increased likelihood of hip replacement in future

Diagnosis and investigations

Hx
- Symptoms present in all forms of JIA:
  - **Joint symptoms** (pain, dysfunction, stiffness), particularly after sleep or prolonged sitting
  - **Persistent joint swelling**, particularly the knee, ankle, wrist and small joints of the hand
  - **Difficulty chewing**, **asymmetric mouth opening** and **micrognathia** (undersized jaw)
  - **Muscle atrophy**
  - **Flexion contracture deformity**
  - **Synovial hypertrophy**
- See above for specific symptoms of each subtype
- Ask about family history

Ex
- Joints may be warm and swollen, but are not erythematous
- Do not miss out the TMJ and spine on examination!
- Look for extra-articular features

Ix

There are no specific tests since JIA is a clinical diagnosis!

- **Blood tests:**
  - **Inflammatory markers** such as CRP and ESR are often raised
  - **Positive ANA** → ↑risk of uveitis
  - **RF positive** in polyarticular RF-positive JIA
  - **HLA-B27** positive in enthesitis-related JIA
- **Imaging:**
  - **X-rays** → usually normal in early JIA but useful to exclude trauma or osteomyelitis
  - **Ultrasound** → may show joint effusion, synovial hypertrophy and erosions (if present)
  - **MRI** → particularly useful for assessing disease activity in patients with long-standing disease and can also be used to assess response to treatment.

DDx

- Septic arthritis
- Osteomyelitis
- Reactive and post-infective arthritis
- Trauma
- Mechanical pain
- Acute rheumatic fever

Clinical facts: General complications of JIA

- **Osteoporosis**
- **Growth restriction** (related to inflammation)
- **Psychosocial, behavioural** and **educational difficulties**
- **Side-effects** of medication

Management

Non-pharmacological management

- **Physiotherapy, hydrotherapy** and **occupational therapy** to maintain function and prevent deformities.
- Encouragement of physical activity.
- Liaison with school is important.

Pharmacological management

- **NSAIDs** for symptomatic relief but avoid aspirin (due to risk of Reye's syndrome).
- **Steroids**: intra-articular steroids for affected joints and topical steroids for eye involvement.
- **Methotrexate**: first-line treatment if multiple joints are affected.
- **Etanercept**: for patients with polyarticular JIA for whom methotrexate has failed.
- **Tocilizumab**: for treatment of systemic JIA when steroids and methotrexate have failed; may be used for polyarticular arthritis.

Surgery

Soft tissue release, osteotomies and **joint replacement** may be helpful.

Self-assessment

A 3 year old girl attends the rheumatology clinic with her parents. Her parents report a presentation of stiffness and limp of several weeks' duration. The onset was insidious and her parents do not recall any specific injury or prior infections. Her parents also mention that one of her knees is swollen and cannot be straightened, but is not particularly painful. No systemic features are reported. Blood tests reveal that she is RF negative and ANA positive.

1. Give 4 differential diagnoses for a child with a limp.
2. What type of JIA is this child most likely to have?
3. Outline a management plan for her.

Answers to self-assessment questions are to be found in *Appendix A*.

Chapter 4

Investigations

4.1	Blood tests	98
4.2	Immunological tests	103
4.3	Synovial fluid analysis	106
4.4	Imaging	108

In rheumatology, investigations can aid diagnosis, predict prognosis, assess disease activity and measure response to treatment. Investigations should only be requested when there are clear indications and results are likely to play a role in shaping the patient's management. Routine blood tests are almost always carried out on patients with suspected rheumatic disease and they consist of **full blood count (FBC)**, **inflammatory markers** and **biochemical tests**.

Full blood count (FBC)

- FBC is the most common blood test used in clinical settings. It is therefore important to be familiar with its practical aspects as well as being able to interpret it.
- It's important to note the normal range of any test is where **95% of the normal healthy population will lie**. This means that there is 5% of the healthy population which will lie outside the 'normal range'.
- Normal ranges may vary depending on **age**, **sex**, **ethnicity** and coexisting medical conditions such as **splenectomy** and **pregnancy**.
- Each report from the laboratory will give the appropriate normal range for age and sex of the patient.
- Ethnicity can affect WBC and platelet count. For Afro-Caribbean or African individuals, the WBC and neutrophil count normal ranges are much lower.

> **OSCE tips:** Venepuncture
>
> - Avoid taking blood samples from the same site as an infusion, in order to avoid haemodilution.
> - Avoid veins that are thrombosed or close to infection sites.
> - Do NOT use the affected arm in mastectomy or stroke.
> - When performing the procedure, do NOT withdraw the plunger on the sample bottles prior to attachment to the needle as this will create a vacuum which may lead to the collapse of the vein.
> - If a blood culture is required, take cultures first before other blood tests. Blood cultures require a top-notch sterile technique to avoid false positive results.

- FBC blood is usually taken by venepuncture, collected in an EDTA bottle, mixed well and analysed by the laboratory within 4 hours from collection.
- FBC test can be divided into three categories (**red cell parameters**, **white cells** and **platelets**).

Red cell parameters

- **Haemoglobin (Hb) concentration** defines whether the patient is anaemic or not. The normal range of Hb for **men is 130–180 g/L** and **115–160 g/L for women**.
- **Mean cell volume (MCV)** defines the type of anaemia: **macrocytic** (high MCV), **normocytic**, or **microcytic** (low MCV). See *Table 4.1.1*.
- **Mean cell haemoglobin (MCH)** indicates iron deficiency anaemia, if low.

Table 4.1.1: Types of anaemia encountered in rheumatology

Type of anaemia	Blood results	Differential diagnosis
Microcytic anaemia	↓ MCV ↓ MCH ↓ Fe ↑ RDW	Peptic ulcer due to NSAIDs or steroids
Macrocytic anaemia	↑ MCV ↓ Folate ↓ Vitamin B$_{12}$	Azathioprine Methotrexate and alcohol consumption Pernicious anaemia
Normocytic anaemia	→ or ↓ Hb → or ↓ MCV ↓ Fe ↑ Ferritin ↓ Erythropoietin	Anaemia of chronic disease e.g. RA and SLE

- **Haematocrit (Hct)**, also known as **packed cell volume (PCV)**, is the volume in percentage (%) of red blood cells in blood (*Fig. 4.1.1*). It is decreased in anaemia.

- **Red cell distribution width (RDW)** measures the range of cell sizes in a sample of blood. Usually red blood cells are a standard size. However, certain disorders (not rheumatological), can cause significant variation in cell size.

Other parameters such as **reticulocytes**, **erythropoietin**, **serum iron (Fe)**, **ferritin** (intracellular protein that stores iron), **folate** and **vitamin B$_{12}$ level** are not part of routine FBC and should be requested if required.

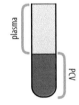

Fig. 4.1.1: Haematocrit or packed cell volume (PCV) illustration.

White cells

Table 4.1.2: White cell count interpretation

	Raised	Decreased
Neutrophils	**Septic arthritis** caused by bacterial infections, **gout and CPPD**, and **systemic cortico-steroids**	**SLE, Felty's syndrome** in RA (rare); **Drug-induced** e.g. DMARDs and **folate deficiency**
Lymphocytes		Common in **SLE**
Eosinophils	**Primary vasculitis**, especially Churg–Strauss syndrome associated with asthma/allergy; **polyarteritis nodosa**	
Other immune cell counts such as monocyte and basophil count are used less in rheumatology		

Platelets

- **Thrombocytosis**: indicates active inflammation e.g. RA.
- **Thrombocytopenia**: can be associated with SLE and RA (Felty's syndrome).

Inflammatory markers

Inflammatory markers are usually raised during the **acute phase response**. Two main inflammatory markers are used in rheumatology:

Erythrocyte sedimentation rate (ESR)

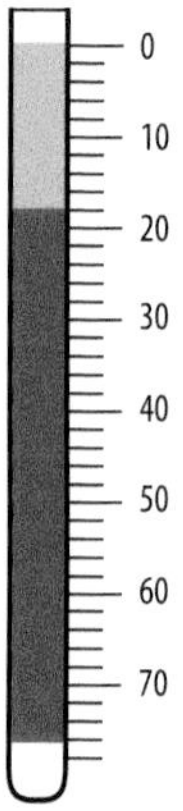

- A **non-specific test**.
- The investigation works by assessing how fast red blood cells fall (due to the gravity and high density of RBCs compared to plasma) through a vertical column of anti-coagulated blood in 1 hour (*Fig. 4.1.2*).
- The rate is measured in **mm/hr** and depends on three factors:
  - **Erythrocytes**: these cells are negatively charged and they tend to repel each other, causing a delay in their settlement. Therefore size, charge and the number of erythrocytes in the blood affect ESR.
  - **Plasma**: fibrinogen and serum immunoglobulins are large macromolecules that tend to get between erythrocytes, reducing the repulsion forces which increase ESR. During inflammation, serum fibrinogen and immunoglobulin increase, causing ESR to rise.
  - **Technical factors**: laboratory technique and delay in analysis.
- In rheumatology, any inflammatory condition, such as **RA**, **GCA** and **PMR**, can cause raised ESR (See *Table 4.1.3* for normal values).
- It is important to note that factors other than inflammation can also result in increased ESR, e.g. **anaemia**, **MI** and **multiple myeloma**.

Fig. 4.1.2: RBCs settle after 1 hour, leaving plasma at the top of the tube. The ESR reading is 18 mm/hour.

Table 4.1.3: Normal ESR range (mm/hr)		
Age	Men	Women
17–50	0–1	0–12
51–60	0–12	0–19
>60	0–14	0–20

C-reactive protein (CRP)

- Any tissue injury or activation of the immune system (e.g. due to an **autoimmune condition or infection**) causes a release of **interleukin-6 (IL-6)**.
- Increases in circulating IL-6 levels stimulate the production and release of CRP and fibrinogen from the liver within **10 hours** of the onset of inflammation (*Fig. 4.1.3*).
- The function of CRP is very similar to immunoglobulins:
  - CRP activates the **complement system** through the classical pathway.
  - CRP acts as an **opsonin** for various pathogens.
- CRP is more useful in **monitoring disease activity** and **measuring response to treatment** than for diagnosis.

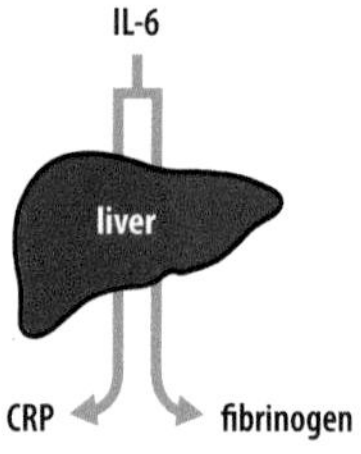

Fig. 4.1.3: CRP release pathway.

Biochemical tests

Biochemical tests are performed in rheumatology for three main reasons:

- To **assess the degree of systemic involvement** e.g. the use of renal function tests in vasculitis.
- To **monitor adverse drug effects** e.g. LFTs in patients prescribed methotrexate.
- To **aid diagnosis of certain conditions** e.g. uric acid measurement in patients with suspected gout.

Liver function tests (LFT)

LFTs are a group of tests that detect any liver damage or disease and they include:

- **Alanine transaminase (ALT), aspartate transaminase (AST)**: increased serum levels may indicate **acute liver damage** (e.g. hepatitis B $\rightarrow$ secondary vasculitis). They can also indicate **drug-induced hepatitis**, mainly dose related (e.g. **steroids**, **methotrexate** and **azathioprine**).
- **Alkaline phosphatase (ALP):** mainly produced by bile duct cells or **osteoblast cells**. In rheumatology, ALP is markedly raised in **Paget's disease** and may also be raised in **rickets / osteomalacia** or **bone cancer**.
- **Albumin and total protein**: **SLE** usually causes a decrease in serum albumin level due to glomerulonephritis. This can easily be detected using urine dipstick.
- Other LFT tests such as bilirubin, gamma-glutamyltransferase (GGT), lactate dehydrogenase (LDH) and prothrombin time (PT) are used to a lesser extent in rheumatology.

Renal function tests (RFT)

- There are two reasons to request renal function tests in rheumatology:
  - To assess the **extent to which rheumatic diseases affect the kidney** (e.g. SLE and vasculitis).
  - To assess and **monitor the nephrotoxic side-effects** of many drugs used in rheumatology.
- The **eGFR (estimated glomerular filtration rate)** is generally considered to be the best index of kidney function.
- EGFR requires 24 hr urine collection and is usually calculated using plasma and urine creatinine level, thus: $P_{CR} \times GFR = U_{CR} \times$ **(urine flow rate)**.
- Measuring **plasma creatinine levels** is an inexpensive, quick and widely used method of assessing renal function. Their measurement is less sensitive than eGFR, however.
- **Plasma urea** and **electrolyte levels** are an alternative way to assess kidney function. However, levels are less sensitive and specific than eGFR and creatinine plasma level, and many other conditions can influence the results.

Uric acid

- 90% of patients with gout have elevated plasma uric acid levels prior to an acute attack of gout.
- It must be noted, however, that plasma uric acid levels may be normal or fall during an acute attack of gout and therefore their diagnostic use in acute gout is limited.
- Plasma uric acid levels are very useful in measuring disease activity and response to treatment in those with chronic gout.
- Elevated uric acid can also occur in healthy individuals.
- Therefore, the **definitive diagnosis** of gout is based on the presence of **uric acid crystals in synovial fluid**.

Bone biochemistry

- There are 3 tests used to assess 3 main rheumatologic bone diseases (osteoporosis, osteomalacia / rickets and Paget's disease; *Table 4.1.4*):
    1. **Bone-specific alkaline phosphatase** – if high, suspect Paget's disease or osteomalacia.
    2. **Calcium and phosphate plasma level** – if low, suspect osteomalacia.
    3. **Vitamin D** – reduced in rickets and osteomalacia.

Table 4.1.4: Interpretation of bone biochemistry in rheumatology

Condition	Calcium	Phosphate	Alkaline phosphatase	Parathyroid hormone
Osteoporosis	Normal	Normal	Normal	Normal
Osteomalacia and rickets	↓	↓	↑	↑
Paget's disease of bone	Normal	Normal	↑	Normal

4.2 Immunological tests

- Immunological tests play a crucial part in rheumatology, both in terms of providing diagnostic and prognostic value.
- It's important to understand the concept of specificity and sensitivity of diagnostic tests, particularly when it comes to immunological tests:
  - **Sensitivity**: the proportion of people that have the disease and test positive for it. For example, if 90% of patients with RA have a positive test for rheumatoid factor (RF), the sensitivity of RF for detecting RA is 90%.
  - **Specificity**: the proportion of people that don't have the disease and test negative for it. For example, if 98% of patients without RA test negative for anti-CCP, then the specificity of anti-CCP for RA is 98%.
- *Table 4.2.1* summarizes the main immunological tests used in rheumatology.

Table 4.2.1: Immunological tests used in rheumatology

Antibody	Clinical use	Sensitivity (%)	Specificity (%)
Rheumatoid factor (RF)	Aids diagnosis and prognosis of **RA**	60–90	70–80
Anti-CCP	Aids diagnosis and prognosis of **RA**	55–80	90–98
c-ANCA	Aids diagnosis and prognosis of **Wegener's granulomatosis**	70–90	99
p-ANCA	Aids diagnosis and prognosis of **microscopic polyangiitis**	40–80	99
Antinuclear antibody (ANA)	Aids diagnosis of **SLE**	93–95	57
Anti-double-stranded DNA (dsDNA)	Aids diagnosis of **SLE** and provides measurement of disease activity	57	97
Anti-topoisomerase (Anti-Scl-70)	Aids diagnosis and prognosis of **systemic scleroderma**	20	97–100
Anti-Jo-1	Aids diagnosis and prognosis of **polymyositis**	20–30	Not available
Anti-centromere antibody (ACA)	Aids diagnosis of limited systemic sclerosis (CREST syndrome)	31	97
Anti-Ro (aka anti-SSA)	Aids diagnosis of Sjögren's syndrome	8–70	87
Anti-La (aka anti-SSB)	Aids diagnosis of Sjögren's syndrome	14–60	94

Rheumatoid factor

- Ordered when patient has any three criteria for RA (*Sec. 2.1*).
- Testing for RF is cheap and **in the presence of appropriate clinical features it supports the diagnosis of RA**.
- It **does NOT provide a definitive diagnosis on its own**: 15–20% of individuals who are seropositive for RF are in fact healthy.
- Other conditions that are seropositive for RF include: **Sjögren's syndrome**, **SLE**, **subacute bacterial endocarditis**, **acute viral infection** and **tuberculosis**.

Anti-cyclic citrullinated peptide (anti-CCP, ACPA) antibodies

- A highly **specific** test (95–98%) for diagnosing RA.
- Excellent in **detecting early disease**; can be positive several years before the onset of RA.
- Testing for anti-CCP is expensive; it **costs more** than twice as much as RF.
- The test has the advantage of diagnosing an atypical presentation of RA.
- The test can be positive in other conditions such as Lyme disease.

Antineutrophil cytoplasmic antibodies (ANCA)

- Aids the diagnosis of specific subtypes of vasculitis:
    - **Wegener's granulomatosis**: antibodies targeted against proteinase 3 (PR3) → ELISA staining will show **c-ANCA pattern** (*Fig. 4.2.1a*).
    - **Microscopic polyangiitis**: antibodies targeted against myeloperoxidase (MPO) → ELISA staining will show **p-ANCA pattern** (*Fig. 4.2.1b*).
- A rise in ANCA can indicate relapse of the condition.
- Other conditions associated with ANCA are **Churg–Strauss syndrome** and **anti-GBM disease**.

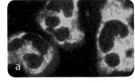

Antinuclear antibodies (ANA)

- There are many subtypes of ANA antibodies including **anti-dsDNA**, **anti-Scl-70**, **anti-Smith**, **anti-Jo-1** and **anti-Ro** autoantibodies.
- The ANA test is a generic test looking for any positive subtypes. Further tests might be required to confirm the presence of a particular subtype.

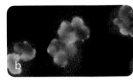

Fig. 4.2.1: **(a)** cytoplasmic (c-ANCA); **(b)** perinuclear (p-ANCA).

- It is the most **sensitive** test (up to 95%) to establish the diagnosis of SLE **in the presence of a typical SLE clinical picture**.
- The ANA test has **low specificity** (57%) for SLE; therefore it should only be ordered when the patient fulfils at least **three clinical criteria for SLE** (*Table 2.12.1*).
- Can be positive in healthy individuals as well as other conditions such as infection (Epstein–Barr virus and viral hepatitis) and neoplastic disease (leukaemia, lymphoma and melanoma).

- ANA can be useful in diagnosing other conditions such as **systemic sclerosis**, with a sensitivity of 85% and a specificity of 54% for picking up the condition.
- Results are reported in titre (e.g. 1:40, 1:60); the higher the titre, the more positive the test is.
- Seropositive results will require further investigation, especially anti-dsDNA test to confirm diagnosis of SLE.

Anti-double-stranded DNA (anti-dsDNA)

- Highly associated with SLE; has a **sensitivity of 57%** and a **specificity of 97%**.
- Can (very rarely) be positive in other autoimmune conditions such as **RA**, **Sjögren's syndrome**, **chronic active hepatitis**, **uveitis** and **Graves' disease**.

Anti-Jo-1

- Although they are classified as ANAs, they are usually located in the cytoplasm.
- Commonly found in patients with **idiopathic inflammatory myopathies**.
- Found in 20–30% of patients with polymyositis, often in conjunction with **interstitial lung disease** (60–70%).

Anti-topoisomerase (anti-Scl-70)

- Very practical in diagnosing and predicting the prognosis of **systemic sclerosis**, especially in **diffuse disease**.
- Usually associated with **lung fibrosis** and **renal disease** in systemic sclerosis.
- **Limited disease (CREST syndrome)** is more closely associated with **anti-centromere antibody (ACA)**, with sensitivity and specificity of 31% and 97%, respectively.

Anti-Ro (anti-SSA) and anti-La (anti-SSB)

- Associated with increased severity in **primary Sjögren's**.
- Can also be positive in other conditions such as **SLE** and **neonatal lupus**.

Synovial fluid analysis

Synovial fluid consists of a transudate of plasma from synovial blood vessels, supplemented with saccharide-rich molecules. The function of synovial fluid is to provide nutrients to the cartilage and to act as a lubricant.

Arthrocentesis (joint aspiration)

- Fluid is collected by needle aspiration.
- Normal fluid will not clot; however, fluid from a diseased joint may contain fibrinogen, causing it to clot.
- An ethylenediaminetetraacetic acid (EDTA) tube is used to collect fluid for cell count, a heparinized tube for chemical and immunological tests, and a sterile tube for microbiological testing and crystal examination.
- Indications, contraindications and complications are summarized in *Table 4.3.1*.

Characteristics of normal synovial fluid

- An ultra-filtrate of plasma which is clear and transparent (*Fig. 4.3.1*).
- Absence of clotting factors.
- Viscous fluid.
- Absence of inflammatory cells.
- Lack of particulates (small particles).

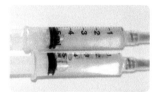

Fig. 4.3.1: (Top) yellow opaque synovial fluid; (Bottom) normal synovial fluid (see *Table 4.3.1* for causes).

The synovial fluid examination (*Table 4.3.2*)

- Evaluation of the **appearance of fluid: colour** and **viscosity**.
- **Cell count** for inflammatory and haemorrhagic pathology.
- **Microscopic examination** for particulates:
  - Gout → **monosodium urate crystals** showing **negative birefringence** under polarized light microscopy (*Fig. 4.3.2a*).
  - CPPD → **CPP crystals** showing **positive birefringence under polarized light microscopy** (*Fig. 4.3.2b*).
- **Microbiology tests (Gram stain** and **culture)** for septic arthritis.
- **Chemical laboratory**:
  - **Glucose** → usually decreased in septic arthritis.
  - **Protein** and **LDH** → usually increased in RA, septic arthritis and gout.

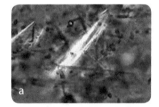

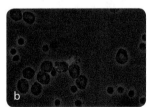

Fig. 4.3.2: (**a**) Needle-shaped monosodium urate crystals; (**b**) rhomboidal CPP crystals.

Table 4.3.1: Indications, contraindications and complications of arthrocentesis

Indications	• To establish the underlying cause of an acute monoarthritis or polyarthritis which include:
	• septic arthritis – which must not be missed as it can lead to irreversible joint destruction
	• other conditions such as crystal arthropathies, rheumatic disorders and haemarthrosis
	• Arthrocentesis is also used to drain large effusions (including septic causes) or haemarthrosis to relieve pain
Contraindications	• Cellulitis
	• Prosthetic joint
	• Patients with coagulopathy or who are on anticoagulants – consider reversing anticoagulation before procedure
Complications	• These include iatrogenic infection, localized trauma, pain, and reaccumulation of the effusion.

Table 4.3.2: Synovial fluid interpretation

Disease	Normal	Non-inflammatory	Inflammatory	Microbial infection	Crystal pathology	Haemorrhagic
		OA	RA, SLE	Septic arthritis	Gout and CPPD	Traumatic injury
Clarity	Transparent	Transparent	Cloudy	Opaque	Cloudy	Bloody
Colour	Clear	Yellow	Yellow	Yellow	Yellow	Red
Viscosity	High	High	Low	Variable	Variable	Variable
WBC count/mm^3	<200	200–2000	2000–10 000	>80 000	Gout: 100–160 000 CPPD: 3 000–100 000	200–2000
Neutrophils (%)	<25	<25	RA 50–75 SLE <25	>90 (if bacterial)	~90	<25
Other features			RA may have decreased levels of glucose. RA and SLE have elevated levels of RF.	Septic arthritis can have decreased levels of glucose.	Presence of CPP or uric acid crystals.	

Imaging

- There are different imaging modalities that can aid clinicians in diagnosing, managing and monitoring rheumatological conditions.
- These imaging modalities include **X-ray**, **ultrasound scan (USS)**, **computed tomography (CT)**, **magnetic resonance imaging (MRI)** and **dual-energy X-ray absorptiometry (DEXA)**.
- It is important to have a framework to work through before requesting imaging.

Before making any **referral request** ask yourself five questions:

1. Has it been done already?
2. Do I have a question the investigation will answer?
3. Do I need it now?
4. Is this the best investigation?
5. Are there any contraindications? (see *OSCE tips*, below)

Once you or your consultant decide to make a referral, make sure you complete a request form to effectively communicate with the imaging department. Ensure the following details are included:

- **Patient's name, d.o.b** and **hospital ID**.
- **Patient's clinical status** and whether it's **urgent** or not.
- **Patient's mobility**: positioning of some imaging techniques require the patient to be mobile.
- **Patient location and travel details**: which ward to escort from and return to, any need to maintain the patient under specific therapy (e.g. oxygen) during the imaging procedure.
- **Contact details**: this includes names (yours and your consultant's), department and telephone / bleep number.
- **Clinical information**: this should show the rationale behind the request, which should include the indications and any contraindications.

OSCE tips: Imaging contraindications

- **Pregnancy and radiation**: any female of childbearing age should be asked whether there is any chance that she could be pregnant and to sign a declaration for this. History of last menstrual cycle must be taken.
- **Intravenous (IV) contrast**: these are nephrotoxic chemicals and therefore renal function tests should be performed before proceeding with imaging that uses IV contrast.
- **Patients can be allergic to IV contrasts**: therefore ask about allergies and previous IV contrast procedure complications (if any).
- **Magnetic resonance imaging**: metallic foreign bodies (FBs) in the orbits, aneurysm clips, pacemakers and cochlear implants.

X-ray

X-rays consist of ionizing radiation that passes through the body and is variably attenuated depending on the structure it passes through:

Air / gas	Fat	Soft tissue or fluid	Bone or calcified structure	Metal

- **Inexpensive** and **readily available**.
- Can show joint damage such as **bone erosion** or **cartilage damage** (joint space narrowing) which can aid the diagnosis of arthritis (see *OSCE tips*, below).
- These changes tend to occur in the **late stages of disease**, however.
- Can be **useful in management**: chest X-ray is recommended before starting methotrexate treatment and requested yearly (depending on symptoms) to check for methotrexate-induced pneumonitis.

OSCE tips: Presenting X-ray checklist!

1. Patient name, gender, d.o.b. and hospital ID
2. Date on which X-ray was taken
3. Comment on the technical aspects:
   - **Orientation** (confirm by the marker (left or right))
   - **X-ray projection**: PA, AP or lateral
   - **Rotation** (if any)
   - **Penetration** (adequate or non-adequate)
4. Describe the visible anatomy **systematically**
5. At the end, summarize the findings in one sentence
6. Offer differential diagnosis

OSCE tips: RA vs OA X-ray changes

RA	OA
Narrowing of joint space	Narrowing of joint space
Periarticular osteopenia	Osteophytes
Juxta-articular bony erosions	Subchondral cysts
Subluxation and gross deformity	Subchondral sclerosis
Periarticular soft tissue swelling	Chondrocalcinosis

Ultrasound scan (USS)

- **A dynamic real-time imaging modality** that utilizes ultrasound (1–15 MHz) as an emission source.
- The ultrasound (US) travels through the body at different velocities (depending on the density) and is reflected.
- The image is constructed based on the amount and timing of the reflected US.
- Widely used in rheumatology for:
  - **detecting synovitis**
  - **detecting joint effusion**

- **assessing cartilage degeneration and bone erosion**
- **assessing blood vessels**: may show vessel oedema in giant cell arteritis
- **guiding joint injection** or **aspiration**.
- **Advantages of US include**: inexpensive, non-invasive, non-radioactive, portable and quick.
- **Disadvantages of US**: operator dependent and interpretation of static image can be difficult.

Computed tomography (CT)

- By using a computer, several X-ray images of the body are taken and converted into a 3D picture.
- Disadvantages: low sensitivity for previewing soft tissue changes and high exposure to ionizing radiation.
- CT scan images can be enhanced using IV contrast agents which are iodine based.
- IV contrast can cause nausea and vomiting, urticaria, renal failure and anaphylaxis.
- **CT is rarely used in rheumatology unless X-ray is unclear and MRI is unavailable**.

Magnetic resonance imaging (MRI)

- Utilizes a magnetic field to align hydrogen nuclei, mainly in the body's water molecules.
- Used in rheumatology for **soft tissue abnormalities** e.g. in **detecting synovitis**, **tenosynovitis**, **tendon rupture** and **intervertebral disc abnormalities**.
- Contraindicated if there is any **metalwork** in the body.
- **Expensive** and access in the NHS is restricted.
- Unlike the CT scanner, the MRI scanner is fully enclosed, which can be problematic for patients with **claustrophobia** or **obesity**.

Dual-energy X-ray absorptiometry (DEXA)

- Measures **bone mineral density (BMD)** in **grams of hydroxyapatite/cm^3**.
- DEXA scan is used to diagnose patients with suspected osteoporosis. Interpretation of the result is explained in *Sec. 2.17*.
- Scanning is most often preferred at the **spine** or **hip**.
- Works by directing two low-energy X-ray beams through the bone being tested. The X-ray is then detected on the other side. The denser the bone, the less the amount of X-ray reaching the detector.

Chapter 5

Pharmacology

5.1	Analgesia	112
5.2	Corticosteroids	116
5.3	Osteoporosis drugs	118
5.4	DMARDs and biological agents	122

5.1 Analgesia

- As with many other specialties, pain control plays a central role in rheumatology.
- The analgesic pain ladder is very useful for determining which analgesic to use (*Fig. 5.1.1*).

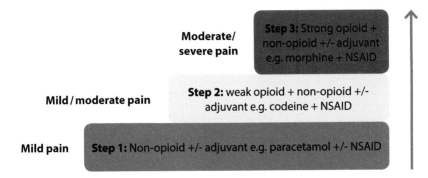

Moderate/severe pain — **Step 3:** Strong opioid + non-opioid +/- adjuvant e.g. morphine + NSAID

Mild/moderate pain — **Step 2:** weak opioid + non-opioid +/- adjuvant e.g. codeine + NSAID

Mild pain — **Step 1:** Non-opioid +/- adjuvant e.g. paracetamol +/- NSAID

Fig. 5.1.1: The WHO stepwise pain ladder.

Paracetamol

- Paracetamol is usually the first-line treatment for mild pain relief and its lack of side-effects and contraindications makes it a very safe agent.

Table 5.1.1: Paracetamol (acetaminophen)

Indications	**Mild/moderate pain** and **fever**
Mechanisms of action	Not entirely understood. Inhibits **cyclooxygenase (COX)** and therefore the formation of **prostaglandins** (similar to NSAIDs but **do not have anti-inflammatory** properties)
Side-effects	**Rare:** rashes, blood disorders (including thrombocytopenia, leucopenia, and neutropenia), hypotension, flushing, tachycardia (on infusion) and liver damage (overdose)
Contraindications	None, but caution in hepatic and renal impairment
Dosage	By mouth, **0.5–1 g every 4–6 hours**, max. 4 g/24 hours
Route	**Oral, rectal** and **IV**

NSAIDs

- Non-steroidal anti-inflammatory drugs (NSAIDs) contain both **analgesic** and **anti-inflammatory** properties and work by inhibiting the production of **prostaglandins** via inhibition of **COX enzyme**.
- NSAIDs vary in their selectivity for inhibiting different types of COX (**COX-1 and COX-2**); selective inhibition of COX-2 is associated with less GI intolerance but they have similar efficacy and cardiovascular risk profile (*Fig. 5.1.2*).

- Examples of **non-selective COX inhibitors** include **ibuprofen** and **diclofenac. Selective COX-2 inhibitors** include **celecoxib** and **meloxicam**.
- **Topical NSAIDs** can be applied directly to the site of pain and inflammation, e.g. in OA. Although they are not as strong as oral NSAIDs, topical NSAIDs do not possess the same systemic side-effects.

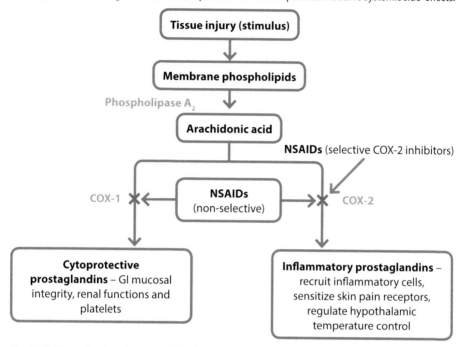

Fig. 5.1.2: The mechanism of action of NSAIDs involves suppression of COX enzymes, resulting in reduced production of prostaglandins from arachidonic acid. This therefore controls inflammation, pain and fever.

Table 5.1.2: NSAIDs	
Examples	• Non-selective – **ibuprofen, diclofenac, naproxen** and **fenoprofen** • Selective – **celecoxib** and **etoricoxib.**
Indications	To reduce mild/moderate pain and inflammation: **inflammatory arthritis (RA, AS, PsA)** and **OA**.
Mechanisms of action	See *Fig. 5.1.2.*
Side-effects	Most commonly **GI disturbances** including discomfort, nausea, diarrhoea, and occasionally GI bleeding and ulceration occur; ↑ risk of CVD, hypersensitivity reactions, headache, dizziness, nervousness, depression, drowsiness, insomnia, vertigo, hearing disturbances, worsening of asthma and renal failure.
Contraindications	Acute renal failure (ARF), chronic renal failure (CRF), ischaemic heart disease (IHD), congestive cardiac failure (CCF), asthma, pregnancy, breastfeeding, elderly and coagulopathies.

Table 5.1.2: NSAIDs *(continued)*	
Dose	• **Ibuprofen**: initially 300–400 mg 3–4 times daily; max. 2.4 g daily • **Naproxen**: 0.5–1 g daily in 1–2 divided doses • **Diclofenac**: 75–150 mg daily in 2–3 divided doses
Route	• **Ibuprofen**: oral and topical • **Naproxen**: oral • **Diclofenac**: oral, rectal, intramuscular (IM), IV, topical

DO:	DO NOT:
• Consider renal function before placing an elderly patient on NSAIDs. • Give gastric protection in the form of a PPI or H$_2$ antagonist if patient is on long-term non-selective NSAIDs. • Tell the patient it may take several weeks for a good NSAID effect.	• Assume that if one NSAID is ineffective, others will be too. Try another class if one doesn't work.

Opioids

- Opioid analgesics are used to relieve **moderate to severe pain**.
- **Compound analgesics**, e.g. **co-codamol** and **co-dydramol**, are a combination of first-step analgesics (paracetamol) and a weak opioid (codeine).
- Repeated administration may cause dependence and tolerance, but this is no deterrent in the control of pain in terminal illness.
- When starting strong opioid treatment, e.g. morphine, opioid-induced nausea often responds well to anti-emetic treatment; this should therefore be considered as prophylaxis against nausea.

Table 5.1.3: Opioids	
Examples	**Codeine phosphate** (mild / moderate pain), **tramadol hydrochloride** (moderate pain / severe pain), **morphine salts, fentanyl, diamorphine** and **hydrochloride** (severe pain).
Indications	**Mild–severe pain**
Mechanism of action	Opioids exert their effects through binding to **opioid receptors – μ** (particularly), **δ** and **κ** within the **central and peripheral nervous system** to reduce the excitability of neurons and therefore pain.
Side-effects	The most common side-effects include nausea and vomiting (particularly in initial stages), constipation, dry mouth, and biliary spasm; larger doses produce muscle rigidity, hypotension, **respiratory depression** (most severe symptom) and confusion.

Table 5.1.3: Opioids *(continued)*

Contraindications	Acute respiratory depression, paralytic ileus, raised intracranial pressure and in head injury, comatose patients, hepatic impairment, renal impairment, pregnancy and breastfeeding. Driving should be avoided.
Dose (oral)	• **Codeine phosphate**: **30–60 mg every 4 hours** when necessary, to a max. of 240 mg daily • **Co-codamol**: 30 mg (codeine)/500 mg (paracetamol) or 8/500 mg: 2 tablets every 6 hours with a maximum of 8 tablets per day • **Dihydrocodeine phosphate**: 30 mg every 4–6 hours when necessary • **Tramadol hydrochloride**: 50–100 mg every 4 hours • **Morphine salts**: see the *BNF*
Routes	• **Codeine phosphate**: oral, IM • **Dihydrocodeine phosphate**: oral, subcutaneous (SC) or IM • **Tramadol hydrochloride**: oral, IM or IV • **Morphine salts**: oral, rectal, IM, SC or IV

DO:	DO NOT:
• Coprescribe a prophylactic anti-emetic when prescribing strong opioids such as morphine.	• Fail to recognize signs of opioid-induced toxicity: pinpoint pupils, bradycardia, poor respiratory effort and stridor. Stop opioid and give naloxone if this happens.

Corticosteroids

- Corticosteroids have both **immunosuppressive** and **anti-inflammatory** properties.
- **Prednisolone** is the most commonly used corticosteroid for treating rheumatic disease.
- Corticosteroids (particularly systemic ones) come with a great number of adverse effects.
- **Systemic corticosteroids** are the treatment of choice for **GCA** and **PMR**. Here the aim is to control the disease by maintaining a high steroid dose for a period of time. Subsequently, the dose may be tapered further with a view to stopping altogether if remission has been achieved and sustained.
- **Local steroid injections** can be given for **soft-tissue inflammation** and **OA**.
- **Steroid-sparing agents** (e.g. **azathioprine** or **methotrexate**) are commonly given with steroids to allow for the dose of steroids to be reduced.

Table 5.2.1: Corticosteroids

Examples	**Cortisone, prednisolone** and **hydrocortisone**.
Indications	**PMR, GCA, vasculitis, PM** and **DM, SLE**, and **RA**.
Mechanism of action	**Anti-inflammatory effects** – via the blockage of inflammatory mediators (such as prostaglandins); **immunosuppressive effects** – suppress delayed hypersensitivity reactions (by directly inhibiting T-lymphocytes); **anti-proliferative (anti-mitotic) effects** – inhibit DNA synthesis and epidermal cell division; and **vasoconstrictive effects** – inhibit the action of histamine and other vasoconstrictive mediators, and also directly affect vascular endothelial cells.
Side-effects (**'CUSHINGOID FAM'**)	Cushing's syndrome, Cataracts, Ulcers (peptic), Skin (striae, thinning, bruising), Hypertension, Infections, Necrosis, Growth restriction (children), Osteoporosis, Obesity (central), Immunosuppression, Diabetes, Fluid retention, Acute pancreatitis and Myopathy.
Contraindications	Systemic infection, liver failure, renal failure, heart failure, acute pancreatitis, diabetes, Cushing's syndrome, peptic ulcers, osteoporosis, hypertension, pregnancy, breastfeeding, elderly and children.
Doses (oral prednisolone)	Depends on route and indication. The *BNF* guide recommends: • **RA**: 7.5 mg/daily. • **PMR**: 10–15 mg/daily. Continued until disease activity is controlled, and then doses are gradually reduced to a 7.5–10 mg/daily maintenance. • **GCA**: 40–60 mg/daily gradually reduced to 7.5–10 mg/daily for maintenance. • **Polyarteritis nodosa and PM**: 60 mg/day (initially), then reduced to a maintenance dose of 10–15 mg/daily. • **SLE**: 60 mg/day (initially), then reduced to a maintenance dose of 10–15 mg/daily.
Route	• Prednisolone: oral, IM. • Hydrocortisone: oral, IM and IV.

DO:	DO NOT:
• Prescribe a **bisphosphonate**, e.g. alendronic acid, if on >7.5 mg oral steroids (long-term) to prevent glucocorticoid-induced osteoporosis. • Give **gastroprotection**, e.g. PPI, for those on long-term corticosteroids. • Give higher maintenance doses during times of concomitant illness and stress (e.g. surgery).	• Prescribe oral steroids for chronic pain syndromes, or vague aches and pains. • Prescribe oral steroids if 'all else has failed'. • Stop long-term steroids suddenly.

- Pharmacological agents for osteoporosis are given either to prevent fractures (**primary prevention**) in individuals who are at high risk of fractures, or to prevent further fractures in those who have already had a fracture (**secondary prevention**).
- Osteoporosis agents can be divided into **bone-forming agents, anti-resorptive agents** or **dual agents** (which do both) (*Fig. 5.3.1*).
- **Bisphosphonates** are usually first-line agents in osteoporosis patients but other effective agents are also available: **raloxifene**, **strontium ranelate**, **teriparatide** and **denosumab**.

Table 5.3.1: Bisphosphonates	
Examples	**Alendronic acid** (alendronate), **ibandronic acid** (ibandronate), **risedronate sodium, zoledronic acid** (zoledronate).
Indications	Osteoporosis (first-line), Paget's disease and bone metastases.
Mechanism of action	**Bisphosphonates inhibit osteoclast action.** They impair the ability of the osteoclasts to form the ruffled border and adhere to the bony surface. They also reduce the activity of osteoclasts by decreasing osteoclast progenitor development and recruitment, and by promoting osteoclast apoptosis, thus inhibiting bone resorption. **Bisphosphonates decrease the risk of vertebral and non-vertebral fractures.**
Side-effects	Oesophageal reactions (ulcers, stricture and erosions, and oesophagitis), abdominal pain and distension, dyspepsia, regurgitation and osteonecrosis of the jaw (rare).
Contraindications	Dysphagia, achalasia, stricture, pregnancy, breastfeeding, hypocalcaemia, GI ulceration, inflammation or bleeding, and renal impairment.
Dose	• **Alendronic acid**: 10 mg/daily or 70 mg/weekly PO. • **Ibandronic acid**: 150 mg/month PO or 3 mg/3 month IV. • **Risedronate sodium**: for Paget's disease of bone, 30 mg daily for 2 months; may be repeated if necessary after at least 2 months. For osteoporosis, 5 mg/daily or 35 mg/weekly. • **Zoledronic acid**: for Paget's disease, 5 mg IV as a single dose over ≥15 minutes. For osteoporosis, 5 mg IV over ≥15 minutes once a year.
Route	Oral and IV.

Table 5.3.2: Selective oestrogen receptor modulators (raloxifene)

Indications	**Post-menopausal osteoporosis.**
Mechanism of action	Raloxifene is a **partial oestrogen receptor agonist**. Since oestrogen inhibits osteoclasts, **raloxifene inhibits osteoclast functioning** and as a result inhibits bone resorption. It is particularly effective in **preventing vertebral fractures**.
Side-effects	**Hot flushes, leg cramps, peripheral oedema, influenza-like symptoms**; less commonly venous thromboembolism (VTE), thrombophlebitis; rarely rashes, GI disturbances, hypertension, arterial thromboembolism, headache, breast discomfort and thrombocytopenia.
Contraindications	Breast and endometrial cancer, history of VTE, coagulopathies, hepatic or renal impairment, breastfeeding and pregnancy.
Dose	60 mg/daily
Route	Oral

Table 5.3.3: Strontium ranelate

Indications	In osteoporosis, a useful alternative to oral bisphosphonates especially in the frail elderly who have difficulty in complying with the dose regimen.
Mechanism of action	Uncertain, but it is thought to have a **biological dual mode of action** by **increasing both bone formation and reducing bone resorption** by stimulating osteoblasts and inhibiting osteoclasts. It **reduces the risk of vertebral and non-vertebral fractures**.
Side-effects	**VTE***, nausea, diarrhoea, myocardial infarction, headache, dermatitis, eczema; very rarely hypersensitivity reactions, including rash, pruritus, urticaria, and angioedema.
Contraindications	Current or previous venous thromboembolic event, ischaemic heart disease, peripheral arterial disease, or cerebrovascular disease; uncontrolled hypertension; temporary or prolonged immobilization.
Dose	2 g once daily in water, preferably at bedtime.
Route	Oral

*VTE side-effect greatly limits the use of strontium ranelate for treatment of osteoporosis.

Table 5.3.4: Recombinant parathyroid peptide analogue (teriparatide)

Indications	Indicated for severe osteoporosis or for women who are intolerant of, or fail to respond to bisphosphonates.
Mechanism of action	**Teriparatide stimulates osteoblast function**, ↑ calcium absorption, and ↑ renal tubular reabsorption of calcium. These effects result in ↑ **bone mineral density, bone mass, and strength**.
Side-effects	GI disorders (nausea and reflux), palpitations, dyspnoea, headache, fatigue, asthenia (weakness), depression, dizziness, vertigo, anaemia, increased sweating, muscle cramps, hypercalcaemia, injection-site reactions.
Contraindications	Pre-existing hypercalcaemia, skeletal malignancies or bone metastases, metabolic bone diseases (including Paget's disease and hyperparathyroidism), unexplained raised ALP, previous radiation therapy to the skeleton.
Dose	20 mg daily (max. duration of treatment 24 months).
Route	SC

Table 5.3.5: RANK-L inhibitor (denosumab)

Indications	**Osteoporosis** (for those who are unable to comply with the special instructions for administering bisphosphonates, or have intolerance / contraindications) and **bone metastases**.
Mechanism of action	Denosumab is a **human monoclonal antibody** that binds the cytokine **RANK-L** (receptor activator of NFκB ligand), an essential factor initiating bone turnover. **RANK-L inhibition blocks osteoclast maturation, function and survival, thus reducing bone resorption**.
Side-effects	Diarrhoea, constipation, infection, pain in extremity, sciatica, hypocalcaemia (fatal cases reported), hypophosphataemia, less commonly cellulitis; rarely osteonecrosis of the jaw, atypical femoral fractures.
Contraindications	Renal impairment, pregnancy and breastfeeding.
Dose	For osteoporosis: 60 mg/6 months.
Route	SC

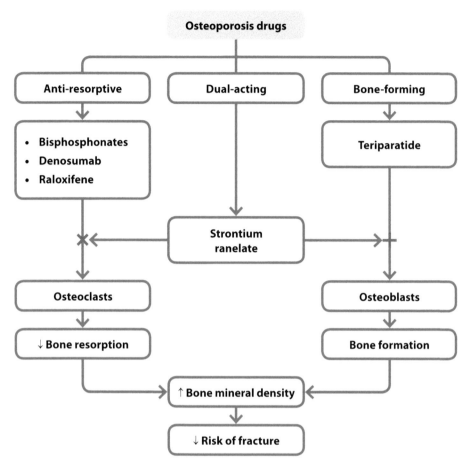

Fig. 5.3.1: Overview of the mechanism of actions of osteoporotic drugs.

- **Disease-modifying antirheumatic drugs (DMARDs)** are a class of drugs commonly used to slow the disease progression of **inflammatory arthritides** such as **RA**, **AS**, **PsA**, and **SLE**.
- DMARDs improve and control symptoms whilst also **delaying progression of disease** and **improving** the **extra-articular manifestations**.
- Early use of DMARDs has been recommended – once RA has been diagnosed, DMARDs should be started.
- **Methotrexate**, **sulfasalazine** or **hydroxychloroquine** are usually used first-line.
- **Azathioprine**, **ciclosporin**, **leflunomide** and **mycophenolate mofetil** can be used if the above fail to control disease activity. **Combination therapy** is usually more effective than monotherapy.
- **Bone marrow suppression**, **liver** and **renal toxicity** are the commonest side-effects of DMARDs and therefore **FBC**, **LFTs**, and **U & Es** should be monitored regularly.
- **Biological agents** are used to treat moderate–severe RA that has not responded well to first- or second-line DMARDs.
- In contrast to DMARDs, biological agents are variants of the **endogenous proteins** of the immune system (usually **antibodies**).
- Examples of biological agents include **anti-TNF therapy**, **rituximab** and **tocilizumab**.
- Biological agents are usually administered parenterally, therefore the onset of action is rapid.
- **Inflammatory markers** such as **CRP** should be monitored regularly to evaluate efficacy.

DMARDs

Table 5.4.1: Methotrexate	
Indications	**Inflammatory arthritis**, **connective tissue disease**, **vasculitis**, **GCA** and **PMR**.
Mechanism of action	• Inhibition of enzymes involved in purine metabolism, leading to accumulation of **adenosine**. Adenosine interacts with receptors on inflammatory and immune cells to regulate their function. • Methotrexate causes **inhibition of T-cell activation** and suppression of intercellular adhesion molecule expression by T-cells. • Methotrexate is **anti-folate** (inhibits **dihydrofolate reductase**) but this is unlikely to contribute to its mechanism of action.
Side-effects	Bone marrow suppression, GI upset (mouth ulcers), hepatotoxicity (cirrhosis) and nephrotoxicity, acute pneumonitis, pulmonary fibrosis or pulmonary oedema, hypersensitivity reactions and increased risk of infection.
Contraindications	Bone marrow dysfunction, immunosuppressed patients, GI dysfunction, hepatic or renal impairment, **pregnancy** (highly teratogenic – requires pre-conception counselling), breastfeeding, patients with ascites or pleural effusions.
Dose	**7.5 mg/weekly**. Adjusted according to response; max. weekly dose 20 mg.
Route	Oral, SC, IM

Table 5.4.2: Sulfasalazine

Indications	**Inflammatory arthritides.**
Mechanisms of action	• Sulfasalazine is a combination of **5-aminosalicylic acid (5-ASA)** and **sulfapyridine**. • Its mechanism of action is not entirely understood but it is thought to **scavenge pro-inflammatory reactive oxygen species**. It also targets T-cells: **inhibits T-cell activation**, **induces T-cell apoptosis** and **inhibits the production of IL-2**.
Side-effects	GI upset (nausea, abdominal pain and vomiting), myelosuppression, hepatitis, rash and reversible hypospermia.
Contraindications	Renal and hepatic impairment, hypersensitivity, porphyria and toddlers (<2 years of age).
Dose	Initially 500 mg/24 hours, increased by 500 mg at intervals of 1 week to a max. of 2–3 g daily in divided doses.
Route	Oral

Table 5.4.3: Hydroxychloroquine

Indications	**RA** and **SLE.**
Mechanism of action	Likely to interfere with the **antigen presentation of B-cells** and **macrophages** by affecting the assembly of **MHC class 2 molecules**.
Side-effects	Visual changes, retinal damage, myelosuppression and skin reactions (rashes, pruritus); ECG changes, convulsions, keratopathy, ototoxicity and hair loss.
Contraindications	Hepatic or renal impairment, epilepsy, myasthenia gravis, psoriasis, porphyria, pregnancy, breastfeeding and elderly.
Dose	200–400 mg daily
Route	Oral

Table 5.4.4: Azathioprine

Indications	**Inflammatory arthritis, connective tissue disease, vasculitis, GCA** and **PMR.**
Mechanism of action	Azathioprine is cleaved to **6-mercaptopurine (6-MP)**. 6-MP functions as an **anti-metabolite** to decrease **DNA** and **RNA synthesis**, therefore causing **immunosuppression**.
Side-effects	Dose-related bone marrow suppression, hypersensitivity reactions, liver impairment, cholestatic jaundice, hair loss, increased susceptibility to infections and colitis in patients also receiving corticosteroids; nausea.
Contraindications	Hypersensitivity, breastfeeding, hepatic or renal impairment, pregnancy, elderly and those who have deficiency in thiopurine methyltransferase (TPMT), the enzyme which eliminates 6-MP.
Dose	1–2.5 mg/kg daily
Route	Oral

Table 5.4.5: Ciclosporin

Indications	**RA** and **seronegative spondyloarthritis.**
Mechanism of action	• Ciclosporin **inhibits early activation of helper T-cells (CD4$^+$)** by **inhibition of the cytokine IL-2**. • Ciclosporin binds to **cyclophilin protein** and the complex then inhibits **calcineurin**, a calcium-dependent enzyme that is important in the regulation of **IL-2 production** by **helper T-cells**.
Side-effects	Nephrotoxic, hypertension, hyperlipidaemia, GI upset, hypertrichosis, gingival hyperplasia and hyperuricaemia.
Contraindications	Porphyria, malignant or refractory hypertension, hepatic or renal impairment, pregnancy and breastfeeding.
Dose	**2.5 mg/kg daily in 2 divided doses**, if necessary increased gradually after 6 weeks; max. 4 mg/kg daily
Route	Oral

Table 5.4.6: Leflunomide

Indications	**RA, PsA**
Mechanism of action	Inhibits **pyrimidine nucleotide synthesis** (and therefore **DNA synthesis**) in **lymphocytes**.
Side-effects	GI upset (nausea, vomiting, diarrhoea and weight loss), respiratory infections, hypertension, headaches, tenosynovitis, alopecia and rash.
Contraindications	Severe immunodeficiency, severe hypoproteinaemia, serious infection, hepatic or renal impairment, pregnancy and breastfeeding, women of childbearing age (unless contraception used – it is teratogenic).
Dose	Initially 100 mg/24 hours for 3 days, then 10–20 mg/24 hours
Route	Oral

Table 5.4.7: Mycophenolate mofetil

Indications	**RA**
Mechanism of action	• Mycophenolate is a prodrug derived from the fungus *Penicillium*. • It inhibits the enzyme **inosine monophosphate dehydrogenase** which is required for **guanosine synthesis**. • It impairs **B- and T-cell proliferation** but spares other rapidly dividing cells (because of the presence of guanosine salvage pathways in other cells).
Side-effects	GI upset (nausea, vomiting, mouth ulcers and weight loss), reversible taste loss, proteinuria and bone marrow suppression.
Contraindications	SLE, hepatic or renal impairment, nephrotoxic medications or gold therapy, pregnancy and allergy to penicillin.
Dose	250–750 mg/24 hours
Route	Oral

Biological agents

Table 5.4.8: Anti-TNF therapy

Examples	**Infliximab**, **etanercept** and **adalimumab**.
Indications	**RA**, **AS** and **PsA**.
Mechanism of action	The pro-inflammatory cytokine TNF-α plays a key role in the pathogenesis of inflammatory arthritis. Blocking the effects of TNF-α results in **reduced inflammation within the joint, reduced angiogenesis** and **reduced joint destruction**. All anti-TNF treatments are more effective if given in **combination** with **methotrexate**.
Side-effects	GI upset (constipation, diarrhoea, dyspepsia, haemorrhage, GORD), renal impairment, hypotension, myocardial or cerebral ischaemia, VTE, rash, fever, seizures, lymphadenopathy and ↑ malignancy risk.
Contraindications	Severe acute infection, immunocompromised, herpes zoster, **possibility of TB**, heart failure, history or development of malignancy, demyelinating disorders, pregnancy (teratogenic) and breastfeeding.
Dose	See *BNF*
Route	IV and SC

Table 5.4.9: Rituximab

Indications	**RA** and **SLE**.
Mechanism of action	Rituximab binds specifically to a **unique cell-surface marker CD20**, which is found on a subset of **B-cells**. B-cells have an important role in RA pathogenesis and **rituximab causes B-cell depletion**, via activation of **complement-mediated B-cell lysis**, initiation of **cell-mediated cytotoxicity via macrophages** and **induction of B-cell apoptosis**.
Side-effects	Infusion reaction, dyspepsia, hypertension, hypotension, rhinitis, sore throat, asthenia, paraesthesia, migraine, arthralgia, muscle spasm and urticaria.
Contraindications	CVD, pregnancy and breastfeeding.
Dose	**1 g, repeated 2 weeks after initial infusion** (in combination with methotrexate)
Route	IV

Table 5.4.10: Tocilizumab

Indications	**RA** and **JRA**.
Mechanism of action	Tocilizumab is a **novel monoclonal antibody** that competitively **inhibits the binding of IL-6 to its receptor** (IL-6R), thereby **inhibiting the action of elevated levels of IL-6 inflammation**, **synovial pannus formation**, and therefore **joint destruction**.
Side-effects	GI (abdominal pain, mouth ulceration, gastritis, raised hepatic transaminases), dizziness, peripheral oedema, hypertension, hypercholesterolaemia, headache, infection, antibody formation, hypersensitivity, leucopenia, neutropenia, rash and pruritus.
Contraindications	Severe active infection, neutropenia, hepatic or renal impairment, pregnancy and breastfeeding.
Dose	• RA: 8 mg/kg/4 weeks • JRA: See *BNF* for children
Route	IV

DO:	DO NOT:
• Monitor DMARD toxicity using the following: **bloods** (FBC, U & Es, LFTs), **urinalysis**, **BP** and **eye examination**. • A **baseline CXR** when prescribing **methotrexate** or **anti-TNF** therapy, to rule out **pulmonary fibrosis** and **TB** respectively. • Give **folic acid** with methotrexate to reduce side-effects. • Consider performing the **TPMT test** before prescribing azathioprine.	• Prescribe methotrexate daily – a common pitfall in prescribing ('M is for Methotrexate is for Monday').

Chapter 6

OSCEs

6.1	History taking	130
6.2	Examination	133
6.3	Differential diagnosis	138

This section is designed to give a brief guideline on how to take a structured history in patients with a suspected rheumatological condition.

- It is important to have a reason behind every question you ask the patient!
- There are three reasons why you would ask a question:
1. **Formulating a diagnosis**
2. **Assessing severity**
3. **Planning investigations and management**

Presenting complaint: ('**Socrates**')

- **S**ite: see *Sec. 6.3*.
- **O**nset: *"How did it start?"*
  - Sudden onset indicates acute pathology such as **septic arthritis**, **reactive arthritis**, acute **gout or CPPD**.
  - Slow and progressive onset indicates **inflammatory arthropathy** (days / weeks) or **degenerative arthritis** (months / years).
- **C**haracter: *"Can you describe the pain to me?"*
- **R**adiation: *"Does the pain move anywhere else?"*
- **A**ssociation: *"Did you notice anything else?"*
  - Pain in another joint (**additive pattern**) is associated with RA.
  - **Swelling** is associated with RA, gout / CPPD, psoriatic arthritis and other inflammatory arthritides.
  - **Redness** can be caused by septic arthritis (redness over a single joint), gout and pseudogout. RA does not cause redness of the joint.
  - **Extra-articular features** such as dry eyes in Sjögren's syndrome (see *Table 6.1.1*).
  - Feeling constantly tired and unwell may be suggestive of fibromyalgia.
  - **Fever** indicates infection e.g. septic arthritis, or an underlying systemic inflammatory condition e.g. SLE.
  - **Weight loss** can occur in RA, PMR and malignancy.
- **T**iming: *"When does it occur?"* *"How long does it last?"* *"How has it changed over time?"*
  - Worse on movement indicates OA.
  - Early morning stiffness which eases with movement indicates RA or AS.
- **E**xacerbating / relieving factors: *"Is there anything that makes it worse / better?"*
  - Relieved by exercise / movement → RA and AS.
  - Pain is worse on movement → OA.
- **S**everity: *"From 1 to 10, 10 being the worst pain you've ever felt, how severe is it?"* *"How is it affecting your life?"* *"Does it wake you up at night?"*

Explore daily living activities. Good screening questions are:

- *"Can you dress yourself completely without difficulty?"*
- *"Can you walk up and down the stairs without any difficulty?"*
- Explore leisure activities and assess the patient's mood.
- Explore occupational activities.

Table 6.1.1: Extra-articular features of rheumatological disorders

Dry eyes	Sjögren's syndrome
Dry mouth	Sjögren's syndrome
Mucocutaneous ulcers	Connective tissue disorders, reactive arthritis and Behçet's disease
Dysphagia	Scleroderma
Headache	GCA
Dyspnoea	DMARDs, interstitial lung diseases secondary to RA, scleroderma or other autoimmune conditions
Photosensitivity	SLE
Fatigue	Long-standing inflammatory and autoimmune conditions
Abdominal pain	Enteropathic spondyloarthropathy (associated with Crohn's and ulcerative colitis disease)
Diarrhoea	Enteropathic spondyloarthropathy (associated with Crohn's and ulcerative colitis disease)

Past medical history

- **Osteoporosis**: any previous fractures?
- **Psoriasis** for psoriatic arthritis.
- **Mouth ulcers or recurrent skin eruption** for connective tissue disorders.
- **Uveitis** for seronegative spondyloarthropathy.
- **Previous recent infections** (upper respiratory, GI and GU infections) for reactive arthritis.
- **Peptic ulcer** when considering NSAIDs.

Drug history and allergies

- Current medication including over-the-counter medication (see *Table 6.1.2*).
- Any drug allergies? If so, what happens when patient develops the allergy?

Table 6.1.2: Specific drugs associated with rheumatological disorders

Steroids	Can cause glucocorticoid-induced osteoporosis. Other side-effects should also be monitored (see *Chapter 5*)
Diuretics	Can cause gout
Minocycline, isoniazid, terbinafine, phenytoin, carbamazepine and sulfasalazine	Can cause drug-induced lupus

Family history

- Ask about any conditions that run in the family, specifically rheumatological conditions such as RA, SLE, AS and nodal OA.
- If there is any family history, ask about the age of onset and prognosis.

Social history

- **Ask about alcohol consumption and smoking:**
  - Alcohol intake is a risk factor for gout.
  - Smoking is a risk factor for osteoporosis.
- **Ask about occupation:**
  - Physical stress on joints (e.g. carpenter) can lead to degenerative arthritis (e.g. OA of the knee).
- **Explore the patient's social status:**
  - Ask about marriage status, family support and living accommodation.
  - Ask about impact of symptoms on their activities of daily living.
  - If the patient is living in two-storey accommodation and has poor mobility, referral to an occupational therapist to assess the situation at the patient's home (holistic approach) may be required.

ICE: ideas, concerns and expectations

- *"Do you have any thoughts as to what might be happening?"*
- *"Is there anything in particular which is concerning you?"*
- *"What were you hoping we could do for you?"*

Examination

This section will cover a useful screening examination known as the GALS: gait, arms, legs and spine. Examination of the hands and wrists will be covered in more detail at the end of the section, since it is a common presentation in rheumatology. Some useful videos are to be found at www.arthritisresearchuk.org/health-professionals-and-students/video-resources/rems.aspx.

The GALS screening examination

Before starting the examination, wash your hands, introduce yourself, explain what you are going to do and obtain consent from the patient. Ensure that the patient is adequately exposed. There are three screening questions that form part of the examination:

1. *"Do you have any pain or stiffness in your muscle joints or back?"*
2. *"Can you dress yourself completely without any difficulties?"*
3. *"Can you walk up and down the stairs without any difficulties?"*

Gait
Ask the patient to walk and look for the following:

- Phases of gait: heel strike, stance, push-off and swing
- Loss of symmetry
- Antalgic (painful) gait
- Use of walking aids
- Difficulty with transfer (sitting and standing from a chair).

Arms
- **Look**
  - Skin: discoloration, nodules, nail signs: **pitting**, **onycholysis** and **hyperkeratosis** all suggest psoriatic arthritis.
  - Muscles: muscle wasting or hypertrophy.
  - Joints: swelling and erythema.
- **Feel**
  - Skin temperature: if skin is warm, this indicates active inflammation or infection.
  - Joint swelling: bony swelling indicates degenerative arthritis; rubbery swelling indicates inflammatory arthritis.
  - Pain on squeezing the MCP joints suggests RA.
- **Move**
  - Assess pronation and supination of the hands by asking the patient to face their palms downwards and upwards, respectively, while elbows are held at the side of their abdomen to exclude any shoulder movement (*Fig. 6.2.1a*).
  - Assess the power grip of each hand by asking the patient to squeeze your finger. Assess pinch grip precision and strength by trying to break the patient's pinch.
  - Ask the patient to flex and extend their wrist, elbow and shoulder.

- Assess shoulder adduction and internal rotation by asking the patient to place their hands behind their back as high as they can (*Fig. 6.2.1b*).
- Assess shoulder external rotation and abduction by asking the patient to place their hands behind their head with elbows as far back as possible (*Fig. 6.2.1c*).

NOTE: When examining the joint movements, look for any discomfort / pain or restrictions.

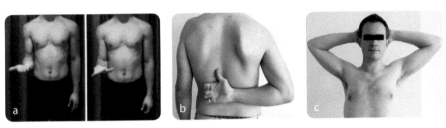

Fig. 6.2.1: **(a)** supination and pronation of the hand; **(b)** shoulder adduction and internal rotation; **(c)** shoulder abduction and external rotation.

Legs

For examination of the legs, the patient should be lying down on a couch.

- **Look**
  - Skin: discoloration, nodules, callosity (thickening of skin, often on the sole of the foot).
  - Muscles: wasting and fasciculation.
  - Joints: swelling, asymmetry and deformity.
- **Feel**
  - Skin: for temperature.
  - Joints: for tenderness (especially along the knee joint margins), warmth and swelling.
- **Move**
  - Ask the patient to bend each knee in turn.
  - Flex and extend the patient's knee with one hand while placing the other hand on the knee joint, in order to feel for any crepitus (*Fig. 6.2.2*).

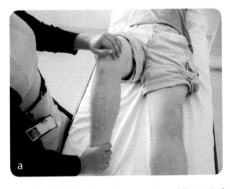
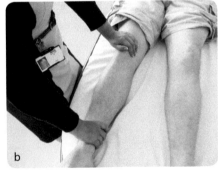

Fig. 6.2.2: Feeling for any knee crepitus while passively flexing **(a)** and extending **(b)** the knee.

- Hold the knee and hip at 90 degrees of flexion and rotate the hip internally and externally (*Fig. 6.2.3*). Keep an eye on the patient's face to elicit any pain or discomfort.

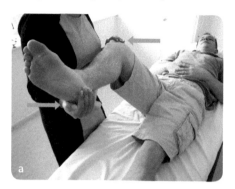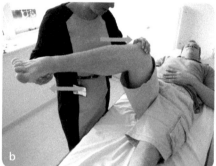

Fig. 6.2.3: **(a)** external rotation of the hip; **(b)** internal rotation of the hip.

Spine

- **Look**
  - Look from the front.
  - Look from the back for normal muscle bulk, to see whether the spine is straight or if there is scoliosis (lateral deviation of the spine).
  - Look from the side for normal cervical lordosis, thoracic kyphosis and lumbar lordosis. Also, look for abnormal kyphosis and fixed flexion deformity.
- **Feel**
  - Feel for any tenderness along the vertebral bodies.
- **Move**
  - Ask the patient to put their ear on their shoulder to elicit lateral flexion of the neck.
  - Ask the patient to flex and extend their neck to elicit normal flexion and extension of the neck.
  - Ask the patient to touch their toes to elicit normal flexion of the lumbar spine.
  - Ask the patient to turn their body on either side to elicit spinal rotation.

Hand and wrist examination

Before examination

Before starting the examination, wash your hands, introduce yourself, explain what you are going to do and obtain consent from the patient. Ensure that the patient's hand, wrist and elbows are exposed adequately.

Look

Start with dorsum then move to the palm and look for any abnormalities, noting whether they are symmetrical or asymmetrical.

- **Nails**
  - Psoriatic changes: pitting, onycholysis, subungual hyperkeratosis.
  - Nail fold vasculitis.
- **Skin**
  - Any scars (e.g. previous carpal tunnel release surgery).
  - Palmar erythema (RA).
  - Bruising and thinning (long-term steroid use).
  - Rheumatoid nodules (especially around the elbows in RA).
- **Joints**
  - Bouchard's nodes (PIP joints) and Heberden's nodes (DIP joints) in OA.
  - Swelling of the MCP joints (RA).
  - Ulnar deviation, swan neck deformity and boutonnière deformity in RA.
- **Muscles and tendons**
  - Look for muscle wasting in thenar and hypothenar prominences of the hand (to elicit nerve damage).
  - Look for prominent extrinsic flexor tendons on the ulnar aspect of the hand (Dupuytren's contracture).

Feel

- Always ask if the patient is in any pain before touching their hands.
- Feel for temperature over the forearm, wrist and MCP joints on both sides.
- Feel for the muscle bulk and any tendon thickening (Dupuytren's contracture).
- Assess nerve sensation by touching the hypothenar (ulnar nerve) and thenar (median nerve) eminences and the dorsal side over the thumb and index, as well as the web space (radial nerve).
- Feel for peripheral pulses.
- Gently squeeze over the MCP joints while watching the patient's face to elicit any pain.
- **Bimanually palpate** any MCP joints that appear to be swollen or tender with the thumbs above and index finger below the MCP joint.
- Both PIP and wrist joints should be palpated in a similar manner.
- Feel the elbow along the ulnar border for any nodules.

Move

- Movement is examined actively and passively.
- Look for limitation of the normal range.
- Assessing power is recommended.

- **Wrist**
  - Flexion and extension (*Fig. 6.2.4*).
  - Ulnar and radial deviation.
  - Pronation and supination.

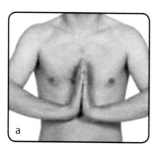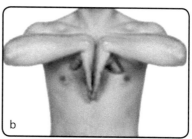

Fig. 6.2.4: **(a)** Excessive wrist extension **(b)** Excessive wrist flexion.

- **Fingers**
  - Flexion and extension: ask the patient to make a fist and open it again.
  - Abduction: ask the patient to spread their fingers out with the palm facing downwards.
  - While in the same position, assess the extensor power by pushing the fingers downwards; this specifically examines the radial nerve.
  - Also assess the power of finger abduction; this specifically examines the ulnar nerve.
- **Thumbs**
  - Flexion
  - Extension
  - Abduction
  - Adduction
  - Opposition
- **Function**
  - Assess hand grip by asking the patient to squeeze your fingers.
  - Assess pencil grip.
  - Ask them to pick up a small object (e.g. a coin).

After examination

- Consider vascular and neurological examinations of the upper limb.
- If appropriate, indicate that you would like to order some tests.
- Ensure the patient is comfortable and offer your help to put clothes back on.
- Offer differential diagnoses.

OSCE tips: Assessing hand movement

- Sometimes it is better to demonstrate movements to the patient, e.g. in elderly individuals who might find it difficult to carry out certain instructions (*"Mr Smith, can you move your thumb like this?"*).
- If the patient's joint is acutely tender, avoid passive movement.
- If there is restriction in range of movement (ROM), find out if this is mild, moderate or severe.
- Find out the cause of the restricted ROM; i.e. whether it is due to **pain or mechanical restriction**.
- Find out if the movement is **restricted passively, actively or both**.
- Pain on active or resisted movement alone indicates tendinopathies.
- When assessing the power, it is best to oppose the patient's movement with the same movement, i.e. if you are assessing index flexion power, oppose the patient's index flexion with your index flexion.

Differential diagnosis

This section will discuss the differential diagnosis of common presentations in rheumatology.

DIP and PIP joint pain

- **Osteoarthritis (OA):** common in females (usually >40 years of age) and presents with bony swellings (more commonly in DIP than PIP joints):
  - DIP: Heberden's nodes
  - PIP: Bouchard's nodes
- **Rheumatoid arthritis (RA):** presents with soft tissue swelling and tenderness that is usually symmetrical (more common in PIP than DIP joints).
- **Spondyloarthropathy** (e.g. psoriatic or reactive arthritis): presents similarly to RA; however, it is usually asymmetrical. Psoriatic arthritis may affect both PIP and DIP joints but characteristically affects the DIP joint.

NOTE: a more common presentation of psoriatic arthritis and reactive arthritis occur in large joints (asymmetrical and oligo-articular).

MCP soft tissue swelling and tenderness

- **RA:** a common presentation of RA, usually in both hands; tenderness can be elicited by gently squeezing the MCP joints.
- **Spondyloarthropathy:** Usually presents asymmetrically with dactylitis (*Box 6.3.1*).

Box 6.3.1: Dactylitis

- Inflammation of the entire digit (either finger or toe)
- Swells up into a sausage shape and can become painful
- Causes of dactylitis include:
  - Spondyloarthropathy (common)
  - Sickle-cell anaemia (usually presents in children >4 years of age)
  - Tuberculosis (rare)
  - Sarcoidosis (rare)

Thumb base pain

- **1st carpometacarpal (CMC) in OA:** common presentation in females aged >40 with an occupational history of repetitive hand movement. Examination reveals bony swellings of the 1st CMC joint.
  - **De Quervain's tenosynovitis:** associated with chronic overuse such as in jobs or hobbies that involve repetitive hand and wrist motions.

Elbow pain

- **Lateral epicondylitis** (tennis elbow): repetitive use of the extensor muscles which are attached to the lateral epicondyle. It presents with tenderness at the lateral epicondyle, which can be exacerbated by extension of the wrist against resistance.
- **Medial epicondylitis** (golfer's elbow): repetitive use of the flexor muscles that are attached to the medial epicondyle. Presents with tenderness at the medial epicondyle, which can be exacerbated by flexion of the wrist against resistance.
- **Olecranon bursitis:** presents with local soft tissue swelling over the olecranon process. Fluctuant swelling is seen in conditions such as overuse or gout.
- **Rheumatoid nodules:** these are similar to bursitis but are **more firm** and are usually located on the ulnar side of the elbow.

Trapezius muscle pain

- Fibromyalgia: associated **widespread pain**, above and below the waist as well as the axial skeletal system, for at least **3 months**.

Thoracic spine pain

- **Ankylosing spondylitis:** usually presents in young men with limited range of movement in the lumbar spine and reduced chest expansion.
- **Osteoporotic vertebral fractures:** usually present in elderly women with dorsal kyphosis.

Lower back pain

Acute

- **Disc prolapse:** usually presents with mechanical back pain and often leads to sciatica (buttock pain and numbness or weakness shooting down the leg and foot).

Chronic

- **Fibromyalgia**.
- If the pain is associated with sciatica, rule out **spinal stenosis**.
- **Osteomalacia / hypovitaminosis D:** usually presents with pathological fractures, and bone pain and tenderness.
- **Ankylosing spondylitis:** presents with dull back pain that radiates to the hip / buttocks); usually associated with stiffness.

Hip pain

- **OA of the hip:** a common cause of chronic hip pain.
- Trochanteric bursitis: presents with lateral hip pain which is very sore to lie on.

Knee pain

Anterior

- **Chondromalacia patellae:** damage to the patella cartilage which usually presents in young individuals engaged in active sports. Pain is typically felt after prolonged sitting.
- **Pre- or infra-patellar bursitis ('housemaid's knee' or 'clergyman's knee'):** anterior swelling and tenderness; common amongst plumbers, cleaners, carpet fitters and any other people who may have to kneel a lot.

Diffuse

- **OA of the knee:** usually presents with crepitus, reduced range of movement and bony swelling (late).
- **RA of the knee:** symmetrical joint pain with swollen, warm and effused joints.
- **Ligament or meniscal injury:** sudden onset and history of recent trauma. Usually presents with locking of the knee.

Foot pain

- **Gout:** acute, asymmetrical, swollen, red joint. Always rule out septic arthritis!
- **OA of the 1st metatarso-phalangeal (MTP) joint:** chronic, bony swelling.
- **Dactylitis:** swelling of the entire toe which can be red and painful. This occurs in spondyloarthropathies.
- **RA:** symmetrical pain of the MTP joints which is accompanied by tenderness and swelling.

Appendix A

Answers to self-assessment questions

2.1 Rheumatoid arthritis

1. Symmetrical joint pain and involvement of MCP joints of the hand are characteristic of rheumatoid arthritis. Her age and gender are also important risk factors for RA.

2. How long has the pain and swelling been present? How has the pain and swelling changed over time? Are the joints stiff? If so, for how long? Is the stiffness worse in the morning? Does it change throughout the day? Is there pain anywhere else? Are any other joints affected?

3. FBC ($\uparrow$ platelet count, $\uparrow$ serum ferritin, anaemia of chronic disease); RF or anti-CCP (+), CRP/ESR ($\uparrow$ during active disease); LFTs and U & Es (usually normal).

4. DMARDs. Methotrexate and sulfasalazine are usually used first-line. Side-effects of methotrexate include bone marrow suppression, GI upset (mouth ulcers), hepatotoxicity (cirrhosis) and nephrotoxicity, acute pneumonitis, pulmonary fibrosis or pulmonary oedema. Side-effects of sulfasalazine are GI upset (nausea, abdominal pain and vomiting), myelosuppression, hepatitis, rash, reversible azoospermia.

5. Measuring CRP and the DAS28 score.

2.2 Osteoarthritis

1. Both hips have reduced joint space, subchondral sclerosis, subchondral cysts and osteophytes. This is indicative of osteoarthritis involving both hip joints.

2. Paracetamol. If this doesn't work, work up the pain ladder (see *Fig. 2.2.5*).

3. Failure of medical therapy and severe impact on the patient's life. Given the patient's age, the most appropriate surgical intervention would be a bilateral total hip replacement.

2.3 Septic arthritis

1. **Look:** signs of erythema, swelling and obvious effusion. **Feel:** tenderness, warmth and effusion. **Move:** marked limitation of movements and inability to bear weight. **Presence of systemic features:** fever, malaise, rash and tachycardia.

2. Gram stain, WCC and culture.

3. *Staphylococcus aureus*.

4. Flucloxacillin (0.5–1 g/6 hours IV for 4–6 weeks).

5. Prosthetic joint, rheumatoid arthritis, diabetes mellitus, low socioeconomic status, extremes of age, intravenous drug use, osteomyelitis, intra-articular injection / aspiration.

2.4 Psoriatic arthritis

1. Nail changes (pitting, onycholysis and hyperkeratosis) and uveitis.

2. **Clinical features:** PsA characteristically involves the DIP joint; RA mainly affects the MCP and PIP joints of the hand (although the PsA rheumatoid pattern presents very similarly). PsA usually involves an asymmetrical large joint, whereas RA presents symmetrically and usually affects the small joints. PsA is not associated with rheumatoid nodules, whereas RA is. PsA commonly presents with dactylitis and enthesitis, RA doesn't. RA and PsA have different extra-articular manifestations.
   Blood tests: PsA is RF and anti-CCP negative, whereas RA is RF and anti-CCP positive.

3. Soft tissue swelling may be the only radiographical finding seen in early disease. Erosion in the DIP joint and periarticular new bone formation, osteolysis and, 'pencil-in-cup' deformity occur in advanced disease.

4. Oral NSAIDs (first-line) and intra-articular corticosteroid injections if NSAIDs are insufficient for pain relief.

5. A DMARD, usually methotrexate. Side-effects are bone marrow suppression, GI upset (mouth ulcers), hepatotoxicity (cirrhosis) and nephrotoxicity; acute pneumonitis, pulmonary fibrosis or pulmonary oedema; hypersensitivity reactions and increased risk of infection.

2.5 Ankylosing spondylitis

1. Given the patient's age and clinical presentation of chronic lower back pain and stiffness which is particularly worse in the morning (and lasts longer than an hour), a diagnosis of ankylosing spondylitis (AS) is most likely.

2. The modified Schober's test. An inferior mark at the level of the posterior superior iliac spine is drawn and a 10 cm segment above this point is also marked on the patient's back. The increase in distance on maximal forward spinal flexion with locked knees is measured. The measured distance should increase from 10 cm to at least 13.5–15 cm in healthy adults. If it increases less than this, it is indicative of AS.

3. HLA-B27.

4. Early signs include bone erosions, widening of the SI joints and vertebral bodies appear square with shiny corners (Romanus lesions). In the long term, ossification of longitudinal ligaments of the spine (syndesmophytes) occurs, giving it a bamboo spine appearance.

5. See *Table 2.5.2.*

2.6 Reactive arthritis

1. GU chlamydia infection, his age as well as his gender.

2. To look for any keratoderma blennorrhagica of the soles – this is a sign of reactive arthritis.

3. Circinate balanitis.

4. ↑ CRP and ESR; FBC – leukocytosis and thrombocytosis acutely; ANA, RF and anti-CCP (all negative); HLA-B27 (positive in 75%).

5. Rest and splint the affected joint. Give an NSAID for pain and soft tissue inflammation. Tetracycline should be administered if chlamydia infection is implicated.

2.7 Gout

1. Gout, pseudogout, septic arthritis, acute flare of osteoarthritis and cellulitis. Septic arthritis is the most important condition to rule out since failure to treat septic arthritis promptly can result in rapid joint destruction.

2. A single peripheral joint (most commonly the MTP joint of the big toe) which becomes excruciatingly painful (often nocturnal), red, hot and swollen.

3. Obese, male and middle-aged.

4. Under polarized light microscopy, the presence of negatively birefringent monosodium urate (MSU) crystals.

5. Extensive juxta-articular erosions with soft tissue swelling.

6. Main treatments for acute gout: NSAIDs (first-line) e.g. naproxen or colchicine (if NSAIDs are contraindicated) or corticosteroids (if NSAIDs and colchicine are contraindicated). The main side-effects of NSAIDs are GI disturbances including discomfort, nausea, diarrhoea, and occasionally GI bleeding and ulceration. Side-effects of colchicine include nausea, vomiting, and abdominal pain. Corticosteroids have many side-effects ('**CUSHINGOID FAM**')-**C**ushing's syndrome, **C**ataracts, **U**lcers (peptic), **S**kin (striae, thinning, bruising), **H**ypertension, **I**nfections, **N**ecrosis, **G**rowth restriction (children), **O**steoporosis, **O**besity (central), **I**mmunosuppression, **D**iabetes, **F**luid retention, **A**cute pancreatitis and **M**yopathy.

7. Allopurinol: 1–2 weeks after inflammation has settled; titrate the dose until serum uric acid (SUA) level <300 µmol/L. Co-prescribe a low-dose NSAID, or low-dose colchicine, for at least 1 month to prevent acute attacks of gout. Febuxostat is second-line if allopurinol is not tolerated/contraindicated.

2.9 Vasculitis

1. Wegener's granulomatosis.

2. Other signs/symptoms:

Related to the upper airway	Foul-smelling rhinorrhoea, hyposomia, epiphora, scleritis/episcleritis, sinusitis, nasal septal perforation and hoarseness of voice.
Related to the pulmonary airway	Persistent cough (usually unproductive), pyrexia, haemoptysis, dyspnoea and post-obstructive infection.
Related to the kidney	Nephritic syndrome.
Other features	Skin rash (palpable purpura), conjunctival haemorrhages and scleritis.

3. Cyclophosphamide, given in combination with high-dose corticosteroids.

2.10 Giant cell arteritis

1. Giant cell arteritis (GCA).
2. High-dose glucocorticoid: oral prednisolone (40–60 mg).
3. Due to overlapping polymyalgia rheumatica.
4. Erythrocyte sedimentation rate (ESR), plasma viscosity and CRP.
5. No; due to skip lesions, the biopsy may not pick up the inflammation. This occurs in 20–30% of cases and therefore a biopsy should be repeated at different sites.

2.11 Polymyalgia rheumatica

1. Polymyalgia rheumatica. Bilateral pain and stiffness in the shoulder and hip girdles, as well as morning stiffness which improves as the day progresses, are characteristic of PMR. Fatigue, weight loss and fever are also symptoms of PMR.
2. Ask about unilateral headache and tenderness, scalp pain, visual symptoms, and tongue and jaw claudication (to rule out coexisting GCA). Ask about muscle weakness (to rule out polymyositis). Ask about bone pain and tenderness (to rule out osteomalacia). Ask about symptoms and signs of hypothyroidism, e.g. cold intolerance, to exclude hypothyroidism. Ask about involvement of small joints of the hands and symmetrical joint involvement as well as extra-articular features of RA (to rule out rheumatoid arthritis). Ask about loss of appetite and perform systems review (to rule out underlying malignancy).
3. Blood tests: raised ESR >40 mm/hour and CRP in PMR and GCA. Serum protein electrophoresis: measures paraprotein level to exclude multiple myeloma. Thyroid function test to exclude hypothyroidism. Radiography to exclude non-erosive joint disease. Temporal artery biopsy to rule out GCA (if clinically indicated).
4. With oral prednisolone (15–20 mg prednisolone). The dose of prednisolone is reduced slowly for 3–6 months to a low maintenance level which is sustained for a further 6–12 months and gradually reduced over the next 6 months with the view of stopping altogether. A bone protective agent (e.g. bisphosphonate) and gastroprotective agent (e.g. proton pump inhibitor (PPI)) should be used as prophylaxis against the long-term side-effects of corticosteroids.

2.12 Systemic lupus erythematosus

1. Malar and discoid rash.
2. Haemolytic anaemia, leucopenia, lymphopenia and thrombocytopenia.
3. ANA is the most sensitive autoantibody in SLE (>95%) but may be raised in other conditions. Anti-dsDNA autoantibody is the most specific autoantibody to SLE.
4. Anti-dsDNA antibody titres, complement proteins (C3, C4) and ESR levels are the best indicators of disease activity. Other parameters such as BP, urinalysis for casts and protein, FBC, U & Es, LFTs, and CRP can also be used.
5. Advice about sun exposure – if she has sun-induced rashes then she should use sunscreen regularly for about 6 months over the summer. She should be aware that sun exposure may precipitate a flare-up. Smoking cessation if she smokes. Pregnancy should be planned. Risk of problems with pregnancy is greatly reduced if disease is well controlled prior to conception. Her drug therapy should be reviewed before pregnancy. Pills that contain oestrogen may exacerbate lupus disease or thrombosis and she should be aware of this and use with caution. Suggest that barrier methods or progesterone-only contraception are a better alternative. Finally, advise that infections should be treated promptly.

2.13 Polymyositis and dermatomyositis

1. Gottron's papules, Gottron's sign and heliotrope rash.
2. Creatine kinase (CK) and other enzymes including aldolase, serum glutamic-oxaloacetic transaminase (SGOT), serum glutamic-pyruvic transaminase (SGPT), and lactate dehydrogenase (LDH) are usually raised. ESR, plasma viscosity and CRP may be raised in active disease. ANA autoantibodies as a positive ANA finding are found in approximately 60% of patients. Anti-Jo-1 antibodies should also be screened for as these are associated with interstitial lung disease, Raynaud's phenomenon and arthritis.
3. Electromyography and muscle biopsy.
4. Measure CK levels. They should decrease in response to effective treatment.

2.14 Sjögren's syndrome

1. *"Are you suffering from dry eyes?" "Have you noticed any swelling around your cheek?" "Have you noticed any dryness around your vagina?" "Is there pain when you have sexual intercourse?" "Do you have a dry cough?" "Do you find it difficult to swallow?" "Do you have pain in any of your joints?" "Do your hands change colour frequently?"*
2. ANA is positive in approximately 80% of patients with Sjögren's syndrome. ANA is always positive in mixed connective tissue disease and drug-induced lupus erythematosus and almost always positive in SLE (95–100%). ANA is also positive in scleroderma (60–95%), polymyositis / dermatomyositis (49–74%) and RA (40–60%). However, ANA may even be positive in normal individuals too (less than 4%).
3. Anti-Ro (SS-A) and anti-La (SS-B) autoantibodies. They are found in up to 90% of patients with SS.
4. Schirmer's test.
5. For her eye symptoms, artificial tears are first-line. Other treatments for dry eyes include ophthalmic ciclosporin drops, spectacle eye shields and humidifiers. Also, advise patients to take regular breaks while reading. For her symptoms of dry mouth, she should be advised to drink plenty of fluids. Salivary substitutes are first-line but cholinergic drugs such as pilocarpine can be used if salivary substitutes are inadequate.

2.15 Scleroderma

1. Subcutaneous calcinosis.
2. Scleroderma.
3. The extent of skin involvement should be noted. Other signs: hand swelling, reduced range of movement (prayer sign), subcutaneous calcinosis and telangiectasia. If there is foot swelling, prompt CVS examination (heart failure) and kidney function tests (renal impairment) will be required. Interstitial lung disease signs should be looked for.
4. ANA, anti-topoisomerase-1 (Scl 70) antibody, anti-centromere antibody (ACA) or anti-RNA polymerase I and III antibody.
5. Interstitial lung disease. CXR, pulmonary function tests, high resolution CT scan and echocardiogram should be performed.

2.16 Fibromyalgia

1. Fibromyalgia.
2. All negative.

3. Heated pool treatment, exercise programmes (individually tailored exercise programmes which include aerobic training and muscle strengthening), cognitive behavioural therapy (CBT), physiotherapy and psychological support.

4. Paracetamol and codeine for mild pain relief. Tramadol for moderate pain relief.

2.17 Osteoporosis

1. Glucocorticoid-induced osteoporosis. Long-term use of glucocorticoid therapy ↓ osteoblastic activity → ↓ bone formation → osteoporosis.

2. Use of prophylactic bone protective agents such as bisphosphonates.

3. Bisphosphonates e.g. alendronate. Side-effects of bisphosphonates include oesophageal reactions (oesophagitis, oesophageal ulcers, stricture and erosions), abdominal pain and distension, dyspepsia, regurgitation and osteonecrosis of the jaw (rare).

4. Osteopenia of the vertebrae. The bone density of the hip is normal.

5. Oestrogen and FSH to confirm premature ovarian failure. Thyroid function tests to rule out hypothyroidism.

6. Smoking cessation and reduction of alcohol consumption (if indicated), weight-bearing muscle exercises, dietary (adequate calcium and vitamin D) and physiotherapy.

2.18 Paget's disease

1. Middle age (approximately 55), male, Caucasian, family history.

2. Pelvis, spine, skull and femur.

3. Bone deformity and enlargement (particularly affecting the bones mentioned above), increased temperature over affected bones, pathological fractures, secondary osteoarthritis as well as hearing loss and tinnitus.

4. With bisphosphonates (to reduce bone turnover) and analgesics (for bone pain).

5. Alkaline phosphatase level (ALP) – it should decrease in response to bisphosphonates.

3.1 Vitamin D deficiency

1. Rickets.

2. Inadequate vitamin D in her diet as she is exclusively breastfed.

3. Serum calcium (decreased), parathyroid hormone (increased), fasting phosphate (decreased) and ALP (increased).

4. Metaphyseal cupping and flaring, epiphyseal irregularities, widening of the epiphyseal plates.

5. Reassure them that with appropriate vitamin D replacement, her condition can be treated. This will allow her health to progress in terms of gaining weight, growing and walking properly as well as reversing the abnormalities in her legs and wrists.

3.2 Juvenile idiopathic arthritis

1. Transient synovitis of the hip; septic arthritis; JIA; osteomyelitis; slipped upper femoral epiphysis; Perthes' disease.

2. Oligoarthritis JIA.

3. Non-pharmacological: physiotherapy, hydrotherapy and occupational therapy, parent education and liaison with nursery. Pharmacological: NSAID cream. If severe, surgery is an option.

Appendix B

Photograph acknowledgments

Please note that the following images are reproduced under the Creative Commons Attribution Share-Alike License; reproduced from www.wikipedia.com: Figs. 7.2.1(b) and (c), Figs. 7.2.2–7.2.4.

Fig. 2.1.1

Adapted by permission from Macmillan Publishers Ltd: *Nature Reviews Drug Discovery*, 2007; 6(1): 75–92, V. Strand *et al.*, 'Biologic therapies in rheumatology: lessons learned, future directions'.

Fig. 2.1.2 (a) Boutonnière and swan neck deformities

Reprinted from *Pathophysiology*, vol. 12, R. Khurana & S. M. Berney, 'Clinical aspects of rheumatoid arthritis', pp. 153–165, 2005, with permission from Elsevier.

Fig. 2.1.2 (a) Ulnar deformity

Reproduced from www.joint-pain-solutions.com/rheumatoid-arthritis-pictures.html

Fig. 2.1.2 (b)

Courtesy of Dr F. Gaillard, Radiopaedia.org.

Fig. 2.2.1

Adapted by permission from Macmillan Publishers Ltd: *Nature Reviews Drug Discovery*, **4:** pp. 331–344, Heike A. Wieland *et al.*, 'Osteoarthritis - an untreatable disease?' (April 2005).

Fig. 2.2.2

Reproduced from *Ann Rheum Dis* (1999) **58:** 675–678, Colin Alexander, 'Heberden's and Bouchard's nodes', with permission from BMJ Publishing Group Ltd.

Fig. 2.2.3

Reproduced from www.kneeandhip.co.uk/hip/hip-pain/hip-osteoarthritis/

Fig. 2.2.4

Reproduced from http://stemcelldoc.wordpress.com/2011/11/13/kellgren-lawrence-classification-knee-osteoarthritis-classification-and-treatment-options/

Fig. 2.2.6

Reproduced from www.kneeandhip.co.uk/arthritis/default.aspx

Fig. 2.4.1

Reproduced from http://crdq.ca/en/participants/fiches-dermatologiques/psoriatic-arthritis/9/

Fig. 2.4.2

Reproduced with kind permission from Springer Science+Business Media B.V.; *Atlas of Rheumatology* by E. Matteson *et al.*

Fig. 2.4.3

Image © Dr Soumya Chatterjee, reproduced from http://bestpractice.bmj.com/best-practice/monograph/1191/resources/image/bp/6.html

Fig. 2.4.4

Reproduced from www.windsorfoot.com/foot_achilles_problems_windsor.php

Fig. 2.4.5

Reproduced from www.sich.co.uk/hypnotherapy/hypnotherapy-for-psoriasis/

Fig. 2.4.6

Reproduced from *Ann Rheum Dis* (2005) **64:** ii58–ii60 with permission from D. McGonagle

Fig. 2.5.2

Reproduced from www.scielo.br/pdf/rb/v40n1/en_10.pdf

Fig. 2.5.3

Reproduced from www.medicalpicturesinfo.com

Fig. 2.6.2

Reproduced courtesy of Life in the Fast Lane, www.lifeinthefastlane.com

Fig. 2.6.3

Reproduced courtesy of Drs Wiesner and Kaufman, Centers for Disease Control and Prevention.

Fig. 2.7.2 (a)

Reproduced from www.flickr.com – photo by "mobiledoc".

Fig. 2.7.2 (b)

Figure reproduced with permission from Arthritis Research UK (www.arthritisresearchuk. org) from: Roddy E. *Gout: presentation and management in primary care*. Reports on the Rheumatic Diseases (Series 6), Hands On 9. Arthritis Research UK; 2011 Summer

Fig. 2.7.2 (c)

Reproduced from http://hcp.stampoutgout.co.uk/gout-clinical-features/tophi.htm

Fig. 2.7.3

Published with permission from LearningRadiology.com

Fig. 2.8.1 (a)

Reproduced from *Ann Rheum Dis*, 'Chondrocalcinosis and Gitelman's syndrome. A new association? J. C. Cobeta-Garcia *et al*., **57**: 748–749 (1998), with permission from BMJ Publishing Group Ltd.

Fig. 2.8.1 (b)

Reproduced from *Ann Rheum Dis*, 'European League Against Rheumatism recommendations for calcium pyrophosphate deposition. Part I: terminology and diagnosis'. W. Zhang *et al*., **70**(4): 563–570 (2011), with permission from BMJ Publishing Group Ltd.

Fig. 2.9.1

Reproduced from *Arthritis & Rheumatism*, Jennette *et al*., (**65**), 1–11 (2013), with permission from John Wiley & Sons.

Fig. 2.9.2

Reproduced from www.thelancetstudent.com/legacy/2010/11/16/the-lancet-seminar-antiphosholipid-syndrome/

Fig. 2.9.3

Image courtesy of a Vasculitis UK member, www.vasculitis.org.uk

Fig. 2.9.4

Reproduced from *BMJ*, 'ABC of arterial and vascular disease: Vasculitis'. C.O.S. Savage *et al*., **320**, 2000, with permission from BMJ Publishing Group Ltd.

Fig. 2.9.5

Image courtesy of a Vasculitis UK member, www.vasculitis.org.uk

Fig. 2.9.6

Figure reproduced courtesy of Dr Yusuf Yazici.

Fig. 2.10.1

Image reproduced courtesy of Dr G. Pountain and Dr B. Hazleman.

Fig. 2.12.3

Image, showing typical clinical presentation of a malar (butterfly) rash in a 31 year old female patient with SLE, reproduced courtesy of Dr Ina Hadshiew.

Fig. 2.12.4

Image provided by a lupus patient.

Fig. 2.12.5

Reproduced from http://pimaderm.com/Conditions-Treated/Hair-and-nail-conditions

Fig. 2.12.6

Reproduced under the Open Government Licence from www.dwp.gov.uk

Fig. 2.13.2

Reproduced from The Pulse, http://clinicalexamskills.blogspot.co.uk/2010/08/dermatomyositis.html

Fig. 2.13.3

Reproduced from *BMJ*, 'Case reports: A woman with muscles pain, weakness, and macular rash'. A.G. Tristano, 2009, with permission from BMJ Publishing Group Ltd.

Fig. 2.13.4

Reproduced with permission from St John's Institute of Dermatology (King's College), London.

Fig. 2.14.1

Reproduced courtesy of Dr Alfredo Aguirre (School of Dental Medicine, University at Buffalo, The State University of New York).

Fig. 2.14.2

Reproduced from www.eyedocs.co.uk/ophthalmology-learning/articles/cornea/505-schirmers-test

Figs. 2.15.1 (b) and (d)

Reproduced with permission from: Pope J. 'Limited cutaneous systemic sclerosis'. *BMJ Best Practice*. www.bestpractice.bmj.com. Accessed 24 October 2013.

Fig. 2.15.1 (c)

Reproduced from www.raynauds.org.uk/images/stories/PDF/localised08.pdf

Fig. 2.15.1 (e)

Reproduced from www.raynauds.org.uk/raynauds/raynauds

Fig. 2.15.2

Reproduced with permission from www.sclero.org – photo by Hazel McCoy.

Fig. 2.17.2

Reproduced from www.prestonchiropractic.co.uk/doctor/chiropractor/chiropractic-Preston/chiropractic-topics/chiropractic-for-osteoporosis-pain-relief

Fig. 2.17.3

Reproduced from http://emedicalppt.blogspot.co.uk/2011/04/hip-fractures-in-elderly.html

Fig. 2.17.4

Reproduced from www.imageinterpretation.co.uk/wrist.html

Fig. 2.18.2

Reproduced courtesy of Dr C. Restrepo, The Rothman Institute.

Fig. 2.18.3

Reproduced from www.surgicalnotes.co.uk

Fig. 2.18.4

Reproduced courtesy of Dr C. Restrepo, The Rothman Institute.

Fig. 3.1.2

Reproduced with permission from www.childortho.com/deformity_hemi_epiphysiodesis.html

Fig. 3.1.3

Reproduced courtesy of Dr Frank Noyes.

Fig. 4.2.1

Images obtained from the Department of Immunology, Royal Liverpool University Hospital, with permission.

Fig. 4.3.1

Reproduced from the Rheumination blog at http://rheumination.typepad.com

Fig. 4.3.2 (a)

Reproduced from *BMJ*, 'Picture quiz: An acutely swollen knee', R. Maggio *et al.*, **340**: (2010), with permission from BMJ Publishing Group Ltd.

Fig. 4.3.2 (b)

Reproduced courtesy of Dr Ann K. Rosenthal (Medical College of Wisconsin).

Fig. 6.2.1 (a)

Reproduced from http://orthoanswer.org/hand-wrist/fracture-scaphoid/treatment.html

Figs. 6.2.1 (b) and (c); Figs. 6.2.2 and 6.2.3

Reproduced from www.osceskills.com under the terms of the Creative Commons Attribution Share-Alike License.

Note: We are making the following images freely available under the terms of the Creative Commons Attribution Share-Alike License: Figs. 2.1.3, 2.1.4, 2.5.1, the figure illustrating Schober's test, 2.12.2, 2.15.1 (a), 2.16.1, 4.1.1, 4.1.2 and 4.1.3.

Index

Bold indicates main entry

ACE, 72
acromegaly, 39
adalimumab, 12, 26, 29, 126
Adcal, 89
alkaline phosphatase, *see* ALP
allodynia, 73
allopurinol, 37, 39
alopecia, 56, 57, 59, 125
ALP, 81, 82, 83, 84, 89, 101, 120
amaurosisfugax, 48, 49, 50
amenorrhoea, 58, 80
amitriptyline, 75
amyloidosis, 27
ANA, 103
anakinra, 12
anaphylaxis, 110
aneurysm, 46
angiotensin-converting enzyme, *see* ACE
ankylosing spondylitis, 7, 22, **27–30**, 139
anorexia, 20, 45
anti-cardiolipin, 57, 59
anti-centromere antibody, 71
anti-dsDNA, 57, 59, 105
anti-Mi-2, 63
anti-MPO, 46
antinuclear antibody, *see* ANA
antiphospholipid syndrome, 46, **55–60**
anti-PR3, 46
anti-RNA, 71
anti-Ro, 66, 105
anti-Scl-70, 105
anti-Smith, 57
anti-SSA, 105
anti-SSB, 105
anti-TNF, 26, 29, 33, 122, 126, 127
anxiety, 73, 74
apoptosis, 14, 55, 118, 123, 126

arthralgia, 30, 44, 57, 65, 67, 126
arthritis
    juvenile idiopathic (JIA), **91–95**
    juvenile rheumatoid (JRA), *see* JIA
    mutilans, 24
    psoriatic, **23–26**
    reactive, 10, 21, 25, **31–34**, 130
    septic, 19–21, 33, 37, 40, 94, 99, 106, 130
aspirin, 35, 59, 94
asthma, 42, 43, 44, 45, 113
atlanto-axial, 27
azathioprine, 46, 53, 60, 64, 99, 101, 116

Baker's cysts, 10
balanitis, 32
bamboo spine, 28, 29
BASDAI, 30
Bath Ankylosing Spondylitis Disease Activity
    Index, *see* BASDAI
Behçet's disease, 42, 43, 45, 46, 131
beta-lactams, 41
biological agents, 5, 11, 12, 46, 111,
    122–127
birefringent, 36, 39, 40
bisphosphonate, 50, 53, 79, 83, 117, 118,
    119, 120, 121
blepharitis, 66
blood tests, **98–102**
BMI, 77, 87
body mass index, *see* BMI
Bouchard's nodes, 15, 136, 138
boutonnière, 9, 136
bradycardia, 115
bursitis, 14, 15, 21, 25, 139, 140
    infra-patellar, 140
    olecranon, 139
    pre-patellar, 140

calciferol, 90
calcineurin, 124
calcinosis, 69, 70
calcitonin, 79
calcium pyrophosphate disease, *see* CPPD
c-ANCA, 42, 46, 47, 104
candidiasis, 66, 67
capsaicin, 17
carbamazepine, 56, 131
cardiac, 46, 57, 58, 60, 72, 82, 113
CBT, 4, 75
cefotaxime, 21
celecoxib, 113
chlamydia, 31, 32, 33, 34
chondrocalcinosis, 39, 40, 109
chondromalacia patellae, 140
Churg–Strauss syndrome, *see* CSS
ciclosporin, 26, 35, 64, 67, 122, 124
claustrophobia, 110
clergyman's knee, 140
clindamycin, 21
cognitive behavioural therapy, *see* CBT
colchicine, 37, 39, 40
colitis, ulcerative, 131
corticosteroids, 5, 11, 29, 33, 40, 52, 111,
     116, 117
COX enzyme, 112, **113**
CPPD, **39–40**
C-reactive protein, *see* CRP
crepitus, 15, 16, 134, 140
CREST syndrome, 68, 69, 70, 71, 103, 105
Crohn's disease, 131
CRP, 10, 100
CSS, 41, 42, 43, 45, 46
cyclophosphamide, 46, 60, 72
cytomegalovirus, 68
cytotoxic, 56, 61

dactylitis, 22, 24, 25, 32, 93, 138, 140
Disease Activity Score, 11, 12, 13
De Quervain's tenosynovitis, 138
denosumab, 79, 118, 120, 121
dermatomyositis, 7, **61–64**
DEXA scan, 78, **110**

diabetes mellitus, 19, 35, 58, 89
diarrhoea, 22, 45, 57, 58, 72, 79, 113, 119,
     120, 125, 126, 131
diclofenac, 12, 113, 114
diplopia, 48, 49
disease-modifying antirheumatic drugs,
     see DMARDs
DMARDs, 11, 12, 26, **122–127**
Dry eyes, 10, **65–67**, 130, 131
Dry mouth, **65–67**, 114, 131
Dupuytren's contracture, 136
dysmotility, 62, 69, 71
dyspareunia, 65
dyspepsia, 118, 126
dysphagia, 62, 65, 69, 70, 118, 131
dysphonia, 44, 62, 120, 131
dysplasia, 83
dysuria, 34

ECG, 56, 58, 123
echocardiogram, 46, 58, 71
eczema, 119
eGFR, 101
encephalitis, 45
endocarditis, 56, 58, 104
enteropathic, 3, 22, 131
enthesitis, 22, 24, 27, 28, 30, 31, 32, 93
epilepsy, 123
epistaxis, 43, 47
erythema, 20, 36, 40, 45, 57, 62, 133, 136
estimated glomerular filtration rate, *see* eGFR

fasciitis, 22, 31, 32
FBC, 28, 46, 49, 58, 60, 98, 99, 122, 127
femoral, 15, 78, 87, 89, 120
ferritin, 10, 99
fibrinogen, 100, 106
fibrocartilage, 27, 39
fibromyalgia, 3, 7, 53, **73–75**, 130, 139
flucloxacillin, 21
fluoxetine, 75
Fracture Risk Assessment Tool, *see* FRAX
FRAX, 78
full blood count, *see* FBC

gait
    waddling, 87, 88
    see also GALS
GALS, 133
gamma-glutamyltransferase, 101
gastro-oesophageal reflux disease,
    see GORD
GCA, **48–51**, 52, 53
giant cell arteritis, *see* GCA
glomerulonephritis, 42, 44, 46, 101
glucocorticoids, 12, 86
glucose, 106, 107
gold therapy, 125
golimumab, 26, 29
GORD, 69, 70, 126
gout, 3, 7, 20, 21, **35–38**, 101, 130,
    139, 140
granulomas, 48
granulomatosis, **41–43**, 103, 104

HAART, 86
haemarthrosis, 21
haemochromatosis, 39
headache, **48–51**, 79, 113, 119, 127, 131
heart failure, 45, 70, 113, 116, 126, 145
Heberden's nodes, 14, 15
Henoch–Schönlein purpura, *see* HSP
hepatitis, 41, 43, 46, 92, 101, 104, 105,
    122, 123
highly active antiretroviral treatment,
    see HAART
histamine, 116
HIV, 23, 25
HLA, 9, 22, 27, 31, 52, 55, 61, 65, 91–94
HSP, 41, 42, 43, 44, 45
human immunodeficiency virus, *see* HIV
human leucocyte antigen, *see* HLA
hydrocortisone, 116
hyperalgesia, 73
hypercalcaemia, 82, 120
hypercalcinuria, 77
hyperkalaemia, 46
hyperkeratosis, 24, 133, 136
hyperplasia, 14, 15, 124

hypersensitivity, 113, 116, 119, 122, 123,
    124, 127
hypocalcaemia, 87, 88, 118, 120
hypomagnesaemia, 39
hypophosphataemia, 120
hypoproteinaemia, 125
hypospermia, 123
hypotension, 112, 114, 126
hypothyroidism, 39, 53, 74, 78
hypotonia, 87
hypovitaminosis, 86, 139
hypoxia, 70

ibuprofen, 12, 29, 113, 114
immunocompromise, 20, 126
immunodeficiency, 125
infection
    chronic, 16, 20
    acute, 126
    bacterial, 19
    viral, 104
    respiratory, 43
infliximab, 12, 26, 126
insomnia, 73, 113
interleukin, 100
intra-articular, 12, 17, 19, 26, 33, 37, 40,
    60, 94
intra-muscular, 12, 61
iron, 98, 99
ischaemia, 41, 43, 45, 126

Jaccoud's arthropathy, 59
joint
    aspiration, 16, 19–21, 62, **106–107**
    cervical spine, 14, 27
    hip, 13, 14–21, 29, 135, 139
    knee, 13, 14–20
    lumbar, 14, 27, 28, 82, 135, 139
juvenile idiopathic arthritis, **91–95**
juxta-articular, 9, 24, 109

Kawasaki disease, 41, 45
keratoconjunctivitis, 65
keratoderma blennorrhagica, 32, 33

kyphosis, 77, 78, 83, 88, 135
   dorsal, 139
   thoracic, 28, 135

laxatives, 35
laxity, 15, 57
leflunomide, 26, 125
leucocytosis, 32, 46
leucopenia, 46, 56, 58, 112, 127
LFTs, 60, 101, 122, 127
lissamine green test, 66
livedo reticularis, 43, 59
liver function tests, *see* LFTs
Looser zone, 89
lordosis, 28, 135
lumbar
   lordosis, 28, 135
   spine, 14, 27, 28, 82, 135, 139
   spondylosis, 29
lymphoma, 58, 65, 104

macrocytic, 98, 99
macrophage, 8, 123, 126
macular erythema, 62
malaise, 20, 31, 32, 36, 52, 56, 63, 88
malar, 57, 58, 60
malignancies, 120
mastectomy, 98
meningitis, 57
meniscal injury, 140
menorrhagia, 58
methicillin-resistant *Staphylococcus aureus*,
   see MRSA
methotrexate, 12, 26, 33, 46, 53, 60, 72, 94,
   99, 109, 116, **122, 126, 127**
MPA, 41, 43, 44, 103, 104
microscopic polyangiitis, *see* MPA
migraine, 49, 56, 73, 126
miscarriage, 59
monophosphate dehydrogenase, 125
monozygotic, 91
MRSA, 21
myalgia, 44, 56, 57
myasthenia gravis, 123
mycophenolate mofetil, 122, 125

myeloma, 53, 77, 78, 83, 89, 100
myopathy, 62, 63, 87, 116
myositis, 63, 65

naloxone, 115
naproxen, 29, 37, 113, 114
nasolacrimal duct, 43
nasopharyngeal ulceration, 56
necrosis, 42, 47, 58, 116
neoplasm, 29, 104
nephritic syndrome, 44
nephrotic syndrome, 57
nephrotoxic, 101, 108, 122, 124, 125
neuralgia, 49
neutropenia, 112, 127
neutrophils, 99, 107
non-opioid, 112
non-steroidal anti-inflammatory drug,
   see NSAID
NSAID, 17, 37, 112, 114

ocilizumab, 12, 94, 127
oedema, 22, 57, 58, 62, 69, 110, 119,
   122, 127
oesophagitis, 79, 118
oestrogen, 59, 76, 119
onycholysis, 24, 93, 133, 136
opioid, 17, 75, 112, 114, 115
opsonin, 100
orthopaedic, 2, 21
osteoarthritis, **14–18**, 39
osteoblast, 76, 79, 119, 121
osteoclast, 8, 76, 81, 118, 119, 120
osteomalacia, 3, 4, 53, 78, 83, 86, 87, 88, 89,
   101, 102, 139
osteopenic, 78, 79
osteoporosis, 3, 5, **76–80**, 116–121, 131, 132
osteosarcoma, 82
osteotomy, 83
ototoxicity, 123
ovarian failure, premature, 80

Paget's disease, **81–84**
PAN, 41, 42, 43, 99, 116
pancytopenia, 58

paraesthesia, 73, 87, 126
paramyxovirus, 81
paraneoplastic, 71
paraplegia, 82
paraprotein, 53
parathyroid, 78, 79, 86, 102, 120
    hormone, *see* PTH
parotid, 65, 66
PCR, 101
penis, 32, 33
pericardial, 56, 58, 70, 72
pericarditis, 56, 57, 58, 92
periorbital, 62
phenytoin, 56, 131
plantar, 22, 25, 31, 32, 63
PM, 53, **61–64**, 74, 103, 105
PMR, 7, 10, 48, 49, **52–54**, 74
pneumonia, 62
pneumonitis, 109, 122
podagra, 36
polyarteritis nodosa, *see* PAN
polyarthritis, 8, 9, 36, 45, 65
polymerase chain reaction, *see* PCR
polymyalgia rheumatic, *see* PMR
polymyositis, *see* PM
porphyria, 123, 124
post-menopausal, 15, 76, 119
PPI, 17, 37, 53, 72, 114, 117
pregabalin, 75
pregnancy, **59**, 98, 108, 113, 115–127
propylthiouracil, 41
prostaglandin, 112, 113, 116
prostate, 89
prosthetic, 19, 20, 21
proteinuria, 44, 56, 58, 125
proton pump inhibitors, *see* PPI
protozoa, 61
pseudogout, 21, 37, 39, 130
    see also CPPD
psoriasis, **23–26**, 91, 93, 123, 131
psoriatic arthritis, **23–26**
psychosis, 57
PTH, 78, 86, 89
punched-out erosions, 36
pyrexia, 44

quinolones, 41

RA, **8–13**, 19, 138
radius, 76, 88
raloxifene, 79, 118, 119, 121
Raynaud's phenomenon, 57, 58, 63, 67, 68,
    69, 70, 72
renal disease, 58, 71, 72, 86, 105
rheumatoid arthritis, *see* RA
rheumatologist, 2, 11
rhinorrhoea, 43
rickets, 3, **86–89**, 101, 102
rifampicin, 86
Rinne's test, 83
rituximab, 12, 122, 126

sacroiliac (SI)
    joint, 22, 27, 33
    pain, 93
sacroiliitis, 22, 24, 25, 28, 29, 32
saddle nose, 43, 44, 45, 47
Salmonella, 31
sarcoidosis, 67, 79, 138
sciatica, 120, 139
scleritis, 10, 44
sclerodactyly, 69
scleroderma, **68–72**, 103, 131
scleromyxoedema, 71
scoliosis, 135
septic arthritis, **19–21**
sequestosome, 81
sialography, 66
sialometry, 66
sinusitis, 44
Sjögren's syndrome, **65–67**
SLE, **55–60**
smoking, 9–11, 37, 56–59, 77, 79, 132
spine pain, thoracic, 139
spondyloarthritis, 24, 124
spondyloarthropathy, 3, 7, 22, 27, 31, 33,
    131, 138, 140
stiffness,
    hands, 9, 10, 70
    spine, 25, 27, 28, 29, 139
strontium ranelate, 79, 118, 119, 121

sulfasalazine, 12, 26, 33, 56, 122, 123, 131
swan neck deformity, 9, 136
syndesmophytes, 27, 28, 32
synovial fluid, 20, 21, 32, 35, 36, 40, 101, **106, 107**
systemic lupus erythematosus, *see* SLE

tachycardia, 20, 112
tacrolimus, 64
Takayasu's arteritis, 43
tenosynovitis, 110, 125, 138
teratogen, 122, 125, 126
teriparatide, 79, 120, 121
thiazide, 35
thiopurine methyltransferase, *see* TPMT
thrombocytopenia, 46, 56, 58, 59, 100, 112, 119
thrombocytosis, 32, 46, 49, 100
thyroid, 53, 78
T-lymphocyte, 56, 116
TNF-alpha, 91
tocilizumab, 122, 127
TPMT, 124, 127
tramadol, 75, 114, 115
T-score, 78, 80

ulceration, 45, 56, 113, 118, 127
ulcerative colitis, 131
ulnar deviation, 9, 136

ultrasound, 10, 20, 28, 39, 40, 49, 94, 108, 109
urticaria, 110, 119, 126
uveitis, 24, 27, 31, 32, 45, 92, 93, 94, 105, 131

vaginal, 57, 65, 67
vancomycin, 21
vasculitis, 10, **41–47**
venepuncture, 98
vesiculobullous lesion, 45
vestibulocochlear nerve, 82
vitamin D deficiency, **86–90**

warfarin, 59
Weber's test, 83
Wegener's granulomatosis, *see* WG
WG, 41, 43, 103, 104
Wilson's disease, 39

xerophthalmia, 65
xerostomia, 65
X-ray, 2, 25, 40, 89, 94, 109

yellow flag, **74**

zoledronate, 79, 83, 118
zoledronic acid, 118
Z-score, 78
Z-thumb, 9
zygapophyseal joint, 27